EXERCISE FOR SENIOR OVER 60

A simple guide with the necessary knowledge to
carry out physical activity comfortably at home;
starting with aerobic training and then moving on
to exercise for motor flexibility, balance exercise to
increase muscle strength and thus prevent age-
related trauma

[Mary Pauline Heart]

Where appropriate and/or necessary, you must consult a professional (including but not limited to your doctor, attorney, financial advisor or such other professional advisor) before using any of the suggested remedies, techniques, or information in this book.

Upon using the contents and information contained in this book, you agree to hold harmless the Author from and against any damages, costs, and expenses, including any legal fees potentially resulting from the application of any of the information provided by this book. This disclaimer applies to any loss, damages or injury caused by the use and application, whether directly or indirectly, of any advice or information presented, whether for breach of contract, tort, negligence, personal injury, criminal intent, or under any other cause of action.

You agree to accept all risks of using the information presented inside this book.

You agree that by continuing to read this book, where appropriate and/or necessary, you shall consult a professional (including but not limited to your doctor, attorney, or financial advisor or such other advisor as needed) before using any of the suggested remedies, techniques, or information in this book.

TABLE OF CONTENTS

BOOK DESCRIPTION

erforming exercises when you are more than 60 years old can be troublesome particularly with joint inflammation or dementia. Be that as it may, the advantages of practicing your body far eclipses the trouble you might confront on the grounds that activity assists with building balance, support certainty, endurance, and energy. Decreasing the gamble of coronary illness or stroke is likewise one of the advantages. Your wellbeing will for the most part improve as well.

Prior to going through any type of activity, you should address your PCP first, so the activity you pick combined with its force coordinates with your wellness. For the most part, you should accept things. You are simply going to practice your body to stay in shape and not for the Olympics.

Whenever you're more than 60 years, you should participate in light exercises consistently with the goal that you will be physically dynamic. Such light activity includes simply moving as opposed to sitting or resting. You don't consume a lot of energy while doing them.

Assuming you are thinking about what light exercises include, it is simply moving around in your home to do things like cleaning, tidying, making your food, making the bed, standing up, vacuuming, or strolling at a sluggish speed. This light activity ought to work on your flexibility, balance, and work on your strength. This should be done no less than two times every week.

It is prudent to utilize 150 minutes to do reasonably extreme exercises which causes you to inhale quicker than you regularly would, builds your pulse, and by and large causes you to feel hotter. One of the signs to realize that your activity is respectably extraordinary is having the option to talk yet not sing. Such reasonably extraordinary exercises incorporate water aerobics, riding your bicycle, climbing, strolling considering your wellbeing, playing tennis, pushing things, and so on. 75 minutes of vivaciously serious exercises week by week are additionally encouraged to be finished.

Exercises that cause you to inhale quickly and hard are energetically serious. It is difficult for you to say in excess of a couple of words without stopping to inhale assuming you are doing this sort of activity. Doing lively extraordinary exercises for 75 minutes can give you medical advantages that are very like that of 150 minutes of reasonably extreme activity. A moderate-power activity can immediately become incredible where endeavors are expanded.

Enthusiastically extreme exercises incorporate football, climbing uphill, swimming for wellness, running, aerobics, hand to hand fighting, tennis, dance for wellness, and so on You can do both decently extreme exercises and enthusiastically serious exercises assuming that you are as of now dynamic. You should attempt to limit the time you spend resting or plunking down. Likewise, reduce the hours you spend not moving and incorporate a few exercises.

In the event that you don't have a decent hold of your feet and you are terrified about falling, exercises that will work on your balance, strength, and flexibility ought to be your center since that will make you more grounded, and it will make you sure.

INTRODUCTION

For better understanding the effect of physical activity on our invulnerability, it is important to realize what physical activity and exercise are. We frequently utilize the terms practice and physical activity conversely, in spite of the fact that there are a few distinctions between them. Between these two terms, there is a little yet urgent distinction. By definition, physical exercise is arranged, organized, and redundant development of different pieces of our body.

In examination, physical activity is the more extensive term alluding to anybody's development. Physical activity prompts physical wellness to have extraordinary significance in the transformative history of people. The human body is intended for activity, which had extraordinary significance in getting food and other important assets, which was unimaginable without performing even hard physical work.

The present industrialized world doesn't expect us to

be in amazing physical condition to get by. We turned out to be less dynamic and embraced a more stationary way of life, which possibly adds to the improvement of numerous ongoing illnesses and the debilitating of the invulnerable framework. Assume we need to keep up with great wellbeing and protection from different sicknesses, not just irresistible illnesses.

All things considered, we should plan moderate exercise or other physical activity meetings something like 3 to 4 times each week. Training is an orderly interaction, and its essential objective is to work on our physical wellness, more elevated level of execution, the working of the resistant framework, and, surprisingly, our psychological state. The exercises performed should be founded on the standard of natural variation. Our body returns to another condition of positive homeostasis.

The most established information on the connection between physical exercise and human wellbeing came from China and India, when researchers and doctors highlighted the connection among wellbeing and physical activity as soon as 6000 years prior. Old European researchers showed the relationship of physical activity with our wellbeing. Hippocrates (460 - 375 BC), in his work "The Regimen," stated, "Eating alone won't keep a man well; he should likewise accept work out. For food and exercise, while having inverse characteristics, yet cooperate to deliver wellbeing."

Galen (Claudius Galenus, 130 - 200 AD) wrote in his work On Hygiene, "The employments of activity, I think, are twofold; one for the departure of the fertilizers, the other for the creation of good state of the firm pieces of the body. Since energetic movement is worked out, it should be that main these three things result from it in the practicing body-hardness of the organs from shared steady loss, increment of the inherent warmth, and sped up development of breath. These are trailed by the wide range of various individual advantages which gather to the body from workout."

Old Greek doctors endorsed practice as one of the treatment strategies to forestall and treat different problems. In the sixteenth century Italy, numerous doctors endorsed practice for youngsters and the older to keep up with great wellbeing and treat different illnesses. In the mid eighteenth century, Ramazzini noticed that stationary specialists experience the ill effects of medical conditions.

Negative practices, for example, smoking, deficient eating regimen and a stationary way of life are the underlying drivers of medical issues, particularly persistent infections, malignant growths, stroke, and diabetes. Do you have at least some ideas that a stationary way of life is answerable for almost 30% of sudden passing in created nations? Epidemiological investigations show that physical activity decreases the quantity of instances of numerous persistent illnesses, including bacterial and viral contaminations and fiery sicknesses, and malignant growth.

Practice immunology is a moderately youthful discipline of general exercise physiology managing the impact of intense and constant physical activity on our safe capacities. Exact epidemiological investigations and lab research started during the eighties of the last century.

Customary 20 minutes moderate physical exercises like energetic strolling, running, or trekking performed three or four times each week have a positive aggregate impact working on invulnerable capacity. It applies to us all, no matter what the condition of our insusceptible framework. It might be ideal assuming you recalled that even a ten-minute workout is superior to nothing is. Body movement, profound breathing, and, surprisingly, light muscle compression is enough for streaming the lymph.

Light exercise advances the progression of lymph and blood, appropriating insusceptible cells and antibodies through our bodies. Hindered breathing, such as during too exhausting activity (low oxygen conveyance to our body cells), harms resistant capacities. Conversely, moderate exercise builds oxygen conveyance and upgrades our resistance since insusceptible framework digestion (creation of antibodies and invulnerable cells) needs a generally high measure of oxygen.

Practice modifies the Immune cell populace and their usefulness in a positive manner and can go about as a trigger of the safe framework. For instance, the convergence of lymphocytes ascends in the circulation system, and regular executioner cells have higher cytotoxicity.

Customary exercise can defer or dial back the maturing cycles of the insusceptible framework. Along these lines physical activity can prompt invulnerable advantages additionally in more established age. In any case, we ought to recollect that too concentrated exercise prompts gloom of certain parts of safe capacity, particularly our gained resistance, and diminishes the customary activity of practically all invulnerable cell types.

In actuality, customary physical activity is useful to wellbeing by decidedly affecting the metabolic state and the invulnerable framework. Moderate exercise strengthens our resistance, both cell and humoral. Notwithstanding, high arduous and escalated practice hurts our body prompting irritation and diseases.

10

CHAPTER 1

WHY PRACTICE PHYSICAL
ACTIVITY IF YOU ARE OVER 60?

The significance of physical activity for our resistance and what changes happen in the invulnerable framework affected by work out.

Would physical activity be able to influence resistant capacity? To comprehend the effect of activity on our resistance, we really want to respond to two central inquiries: How exercise upholds or smothers the insusceptible framework, and what physical activity is best for strengthening your invulnerability? Many examinations exhibit that physical activity seriously affects the insusceptible framework.

We need to recognize intense from ongoing impacts of activity on the number and activity of the insusceptible cells. Significant are factors describing the workout, like kind of activity, now is the right time, and force. Our invulnerable framework reacts diversely to intense and constant exercise.

The moderate aerobic exercise we can treat as an enhancer of different insusceptible boundaries working on our protection from illnesses and contaminations. Interestingly, focused energy physical activity diminishes the invulnerable framework's capacity to battle against attacking microbes and builds the gamble of fostering the sickness.

We as a rule partition the resistant framework into intrinsic and versatile parts relying upon the idea of the invulnerable reaction. We regularly treat stomach and mucosal hindrances capacities and cell resistance independently. In the logical writing, an often-experienced term is gained insusceptibility, which is additionally separated into versatile and aloof invulnerability.

To better understand the effect of physical activity on our resistance, we ought to think about all of the previously mentioned sorts of invulnerable reactions. In any case, we should take note that the terms versatile and gained mean something very similar and allude to a similar piece of the safe framework.

There is general understanding that exercises emphatically or contrarily influence our insusceptibility relying upon their force and span. Ordinary, short enduring (under 40 minutes) moderate power practice helps our opposition against different microbes, while drawn out and serious training contrarily influences our invulnerability.

Moderate power training works on resistant reactions to microorganisms and immunization, brings down different irritations, and works on our invulnerability against malignant growths, cardiovascular illnesses, diabetes, and numerous other unsafe circumstances and illnesses. It has an immune-upgrading impact.

Then again, focused energy demanding activity stifles cell resistance, debilitating reactions to antigens (expanding manifestations of upper respiratory tract diseases, for instance), alleged immunosuppressive impact.

The impacts of activity are mutually dependent on different variables that manage safe capacity, like hereditary profile, natural stressors (allergens, outrageous temperatures), dietary status, and wellbeing problems or illnesses advancing incendiary cycles. Consequently, the above factors, along with weighty effort, lift the gamble of disease.

Normal moderate physical activity upgrades the trading of resistant cells between the blood dissemination framework and the fringe lymphoid framework, and different body tissues. This regular trade of safe cells further develops wellbeing and makes the gamble of infections lower.

Both intense and constant exercise adjusts the number and capacity of invulnerable cells. Transient moderate exercise can upgrade versatile and inborn safe reactions.

Simultaneously, too escalated long-haul training diminishes invulnerable cell capacities and expands immunosuppressive instruments (administrative T cell pathways, for instance).

Insusceptible cells develop, multiply, and produce cytokines because of activity stress. These cycles

14

require supply of an adequate measure of energy through metabolic pathways. Such connections between the two frameworks are apparent during recuperation from high serious training.

Leukocytosis (raised number of white platelets in the circulatory system) during extraordinary physical training affirms that too concentrated exercise is liable for the downturn of the insusceptible framework.

It additionally adds to diminishing proliferative activity and capacity T-lymphocytes, regular executioner cells, and macrophages activity. Moreover, an expansion in the recurrence and profundity of breathing during concentrated practicing prompts parchedness of the mucous films.

Lower mucociliary leeway makes an increment in inclination of upper respiratory lot diseases. Focused energy practice causes different gastrointestinal indications, for example, bulging, sickness, or issues, among others.

The reason for these issues might be diminished penetrability and diminished digestive obstruction work. Expanded digestive penetrability is the reason for expanded vulnerability to immune system illnesses and contamination since microorganisms enter the circulatory system all the more without any problem.

The potential elements influencing the safe framework reaction to the exercises incorporate our age and wellness level, sex, the sort of physical activity, and training load implies force (exertion level) and volume (number of reiteration and term).

Natural resistance and physical activity

The natural resistance that goes with us from birth is the main vague line of protection against harmful microbes. It is not entirely settled. The Innate safe reaction begins rapidly and doesn't need introductory actuation like a procured reaction.

The natural safe framework incorporates physical boundaries like our skin, compound parts like tears, and the supplement framework (proteins intercede phagocytosis and collaborate with antibodies).

The inborn framework incorporates different safe

cells, including macrophages, monocytes, regular executioner cells (perceive changed cells), neutrophils, and others. Physical activity adjusts the number and activity of these cells.

Macrophages. Concentrated, depleting exercise decreases macrophage phagocytic activity that relies upon the activity force. In examination, moderate exercise upgrades macrophage exercises (adherence, phagocytosis), while debilitating activity doesn't influence macrophage usefulness.

Monocytes. Drawn out practice expands the monocyte's phagocytic activity. Monocytes assembled by physical activity move to skeletal muscle and separate into macrophages that assist to fix and recover harmed muscle cells.

Neutrophils. Neutrophils establish close to 60% of coursing leukocytes. They play a fundamental part in guarding against attacking infections and microorganisms, killing them by phagocytosis (ingestion). Practice influences the neutrophils somehow or another. Their phagocytic limit is 70%

17

lower still in prepared people.

Difficult physical activity impedes or drains neutrophil work, making expanded vulnerability disease, while moderate exercise upgrades the activity of neutrophils. Drawn out bad changes in neutrophils capacity and number incline toward different contaminations.

Normal executioner cells. The effect of extreme exercise on the normal executioner cell's capacity is biphasic, beginning upgrade, and postponed concealment. Their cytolytic activity is higher toward the finish of moderate exercise. Useful changes in normal executioner cells' cytotoxicity rely upon the span and force of training.

Moderate exercise significantly builds the quantity of regular executioner cells in the circulation system and advances the rearrangement of normal executioner cells from the blood to different tissues.

The pressure chemical cortisol directs natural resistant cell capacities. Moderate power practice improves invulnerable cell activity and brings down the discharge of cortisol, while an extreme focus workout expands the emission of cortisol and consequently diminishes the activity of safe cells. Catecholamines influence leukocyte numbers and capacities, and concentrated training hoists their level.

Gained invulnerability and physical activity

Inspecting the accessible writing, famous and logical, we can observe the terms versatile or explicit insusceptibility showing equivalent to procured resistance. The primary errand, as intrinsic invulnerability, is to obliterate microbes and intrusive microorganisms.

The obtained insusceptible reaction utilizes T-lymphocytes (produce and delivery cytokines) and B-lymphocytes (produce and delivery antibodies). This insusceptible reaction can separate into a humoral reaction interceded by antibodies and a cell reaction intervened by T-lymphocytes. Ordinary physical activity adjusts the capacity of B and T cells.

The introduction of antigens to T-aide lymphocytes sets off this safeguard component. We partition Tassistant lymphocytes into two fundamental sorts, type 1 (Th1) and type 2 (Th2) cells. This division relies upon the cytokines that they produce and deliver. Interleukins are cytokines that power other safe cells to multiply, develop and separate movement and bond.

Monocytes and macrophages likewise produce and deliver cytokines. Th1 lymphocytes assume a fundamental part in the annihilation of intracellular microbes, for example, infections, while Th2 cells in assurance against extracellular microorganisms and animate the development of antibodies by B-lymphocytes.

Changes in T-cells work are relative to practice power and term. Intense serious exercise instigates transient changes in the quantity of coursing lymphocytes that fall beneath pre-practice levels. After a specific rest time (generally 24 hours), the quantity of lymphocytes gets back to typical levels.

These progressions basically connect with the number of inhabitants in T-cells and B-cells less significantly and are relative to practice power and length. Nonetheless, serious physical activity diminishes the quantity of Th1 cells yet littly affects the quantity of Th2 cells.

Work out instigated diminishes in T-cells work (more modest numbers) may prompt expanded helplessness to viral contaminations. Durable difficult exercise decreases the capacity of T cells to relocate to the tainted destinations.

Intense exercise causes transient changes in the quantity of lymphocytes in the blood.

Mucosal insusceptibility and physical activity

The significant job of the mucosal safe framework is to safeguard surfaces of the wholesome, genitourinary, and respiratory plots against microorganisms (infections, microscopic organisms) attempting to attack our body through mucosal layers. Do you have any idea that the surface region of our mucosa is almost 400 square meters while the outer layer of our skin is 1.8 square meters as it were?

The mucosal resistant framework is the biggest piece

of our insusceptible framework, and we can say that it is the primary line of our guard framework. We can isolate it into uninvolved (physical hindrance) and dynamic (versatile and inborn invulnerable reactions) parts. Physical hindrance and stomach corrosive, bodily fluid emission, and dynamic peristalsis keep microbes from entering our body.

Insusceptible cells in the stomach are put in the alleged lamina propria (a slender layer of connective tissue that structures mucous films). Gatherings of particular lymphoid totals, Peyer's patches, are an assortment of B and T cells put underneath epithelial cells taking an example of little different unfamiliar particles. Do you have at least some ideas that 80% (or a greater amount of) the actuated B-cells are situated in the digestive mucosa?

Enduring serious physical pressure causes changes in the assimilation of supplements and adjustment of reactivity of the mucosal insusceptibility that can prompt a fundamental fiery state, particularly inside respiratory and urinary frameworks, diminishing protection from different bacterial or viral diseases.

Assume you participate in energetic exercise and notice indications like weariness, fever, hack, looseness of the bowels, myalgia, or heaving. All things considered, you should stop your training and take a satisfactory time of rest until referenced side effects vanish.

You should take note that concentrated difficult training could stifle mucosal invulnerability while moderate exercise decidedly influences our mucosal resistant boundary.

Neuroendocrine and metabolic variables

Numerous instruments are fundamental to the connection among practice and the working of the safe framework. Neuroendocrine factors like adrenaline, noradrenaline, cortisol, and development chemicals are among them. During the training meeting, the levels of these chemicals are raised, then, at that point, go down during the rest time frame, and return to pre-practice levels.

Adrenaline and, less significantly, noradrenaline intercede practice impact on lymphocytes elements changing regular executioner cells and T-cells activity. Referenced chemicals likewise increment levels of development chemical and catecholamines, intervening the effect on neutrophils. Cytokines are another physical pressure related variable.

Physical activity changes the digestion of the skeletal muscles. The creation and arrival of glutamine is one significant model here. Glutamine is the amino corrosive with the most elevated fixation in the human body, and it represents more than 60% of all free amino acids.

It is a significant fuel for lymphocytes and macrophages. Skeletal muscle is the essential wellspring of glutamine engaged with its creation and delivery into the circulatory system.

A few specialists propose that skeletal muscle assumes a significant part in glutamine usage by the resistant cells. On account of these cycles, skeletal muscle can impact the insusceptible framework straightforwardly.

During serious physical activity, the interest of muscles and different organs for glutamine increases quickly, which causes the invulnerable framework to feel its absence. It influences the elements of lymphocytes and monocytes. After extreme, enduring physical activity, the glutamine level decreases in the circulatory framework.

Intense, moderate versus constant exercise

The connection between the degree of physical activity and our resistance. Different systems of intense and constant exercise assume explicit parts in adjusting the activity of intrinsic and procured invulnerable reactions. Many investigations show that activity regulates the number and capacity of intrinsic resistant cells. Moderate exercise has gainful results in the avoidance and recovery of numerous different sicknesses.

Physical activity might differ day by day, though wellness remains moderately static. Delayed and concentrated training prompts the arrival of stress chemicals, for example, cortisol and adrenaline that smother the activity of the insusceptible framework. Moderate-force exercises animate cell invulnerability, while concentrated and debilitating workouts, running against the norm, decrease the specific boundaries of the insusceptible reaction.

Each training meeting assembles safe cells and accordingly safeguards us from microbes (microscopic organisms and infections) and forestalls reactivation of the inactive infections. During exercise, skeletal muscle compressions cause emission of the flagging proteins like interleukins that diminish irritation (interleukin-6) and back lymphocyte multiplication (interleukin-7).

Better bloodstream during exercise further develops distribution of the insusceptible cells between the blood and lymphatic vessels and fringe tissues. Indeed, even moderate physical activity invigorates this development. Moreover, exercise can expand the quantity of antibodies after immunization and upgrade the reaction to inoculation.

Escalated, durable training influences versatile safe

framework usefulness just to a little degree contrasted with the response of the natural invulnerable framework. The International Society of Exercise and Immunology (ISEI) states that the insusceptible brokenness after practice is more noticeable while the training is consistently drawn out over 1 hour and performed at moderate to focused energy. Debilitated capacity of the invulnerable framework endures as long as 72 hours.

Malignant growth, sickness, and exercise

Any physical activity can further develop resistance and treatment results in numerous infections no matter what our age. Work out, particularly those rehearsed consistently at low or moderate force, is significantly significant for keeping up with great wellbeing and wellness.

Activity smothers aggravation brought about by numerous ongoing illnesses, for example, cardiovascular illnesses, type-2 diabetes, and a few explicit sorts of malignant growth. Numerous competitors undertaking escalated practice regularly experience the ill effects of gastrointestinal and upper respiratory parcel issues.

The metabolic limit of resistant cells is decreased during the recuperation time frame after difficult physical activity causing transient immunosuppression (the quantities of circling insusceptible cells is lower). This condition can endure up to around 48 hours, during which we are more presented not exclusively to upper respiratory parcel diseases yet additionally to other medical issues.

Most of the top thoroughly prepared competitors frequently have indications of upper respiratory lot diseases. Since essential contaminations are impossible, the main sources are the reactivation of inactive infections and other irritation reasons.

Assuming you give a stationary, dormant way of life, instinctive fat collects somewhat rapidly and initiates provocative pathways. Persistent aggravation prompts atherosclerosis, neurodegenerative illnesses and advances cancer development and numerous different problems related with physical inactivity.

28

Numerous medical advantages of normal exercise with moderate or low power have long haul mitigating and transient strengthening of the safe framework impacts. In malignant growth patient's regular executioner cells activity, lymphocyte multiplication rate, and the quantity of granulocytes expanded.

Ordinary moderate exercise decreases defenselessness to malignant growth while too serious comprehensive training, opposite, expands powerlessness to disease. We should take note that neoplastic changed cells can keep away from obliteration by the debilitated invulnerable framework by an impeded insusceptible reaction to the malignant growth cells.

Standard physical activity lessens the rate of a few kinds of disease like colon, bosom, lung, and pancreatic malignant growths. It has a restorative impact by lessening disease repeat, expanding patient endurance, and working on personal satisfaction.

It is the ideal opportunity for a rundown

We definitely realize that assuming we are all the

more physically dynamic and consistently participate in moderate-force physical exercise, our invulnerable framework works much better. Our protection from contamination and constant sicknesses is better. Indeed, even locally established exercises limit the gamble of getting irresistible infections.

We needn't bother with exercise centers or convoluted gadgets. Any even light physical activity is advantageous for our wellbeing. Albeit numerous experts suggest 160 minutes of activity each week (around 20 minutes per day), even a couple of moments is useful.

The most widely recognized resistant framework

parts and their reaction to physical activity.

The insusceptible framework responds to physical activity as per the strength of physiological pressure and responsibility. We can consider the year 1902 as the beginning of activity immunology when it was observed that the quantity of white platelets in Boston long distance runners rose after the race was done.

The impact of activity on our regular resistance relies essentially upon communications among substantial and autonomic sensory systems and endocrine framework usefulness by reestablishing chemical balance, particularly development of chemical and cortisol. The two chemicals fundamentally affect our resistant framework.

Customary physical activity organizes the activity of each of the three frameworks: substantial, autonomic, and endocrine frameworks. Their reaction turns out to be more coordinated. Interestingly, intense exercise causes extreme changes in the resistant framework that are not useful for our invulnerability. A few significant parts of our resistant framework respond adversely to weighty, dependable effort. Such unfriendly responses happen in the mucosal tissue of the upper respiratory plot, lung, skin, and muscle.

Serious training keeps going one hour or more invigorates the safe framework pointedly yet just before all else. Not many hours subsequent to working out, the insusceptible framework begins to get more fragile. Its capacity to battle against outside trespassers is reducing. In any case, it is an exceptionally individual attribute. This period can last a couple of hours or even an entire day. Hence, arranging of practicing meetings and rest periods is huge, relies upon a singular quality.

CHAPTER 2
THE PHYSICAL ACTIVITY
PROGRAM.

W hat physical activity to pick and what might be best for your way of life. Currently in antiquated times, individuals knew about the advantages of physical activity for our wellbeing. The Athenian logician Plato (424-348 BC) broadcasted that absence of physical activity annihilates great circumstances and wellbeing, and customary exercise permits us to remain solid and fit.

We for the most part characterize physical activity as any development of our body brought about by skeletal muscle constrictions. This classification incorporates sporting exercises (strolling, running, and bicycling), performing physical work, and different family exercises. While working out, we can regard it as a sub-classification of physical activity, and it is purposive, arranged, dull physical development.

For instance, moderate-force energetic strolling brings medical advantages for something like ten minutes (close to 160 minutes per week). We need to recollect that too low physical force is inadequate, and we can say that those individuals are physically dormant.

Notwithstanding, in the event that we supplant our inactive way of life with even light-power physical activity, benefits for our wellbeing will be apparent and certain. Many examinations show connections between a latent, inactive life and expanded helplessness to different constant illnesses.

The World Health Organization says that absence of activity is the fourth significant gamble factor for creating numerous illnesses, the advancement of different diseases, and untimely mortality. Rehearsing exercises changes the physiology of our body and supports our insusceptible framework, and changes our mind, disposition to life, and our whole prosperity.

Different physical activity improves our

insusceptibility and prompts better clinical therapy results of normal infections like disease, cardiovascular, metabolic, and neuro-degenerative problems. Physiological transformation results from standard exercise, and its greatness relies upon the mode, time, and force.

We need to take note that appropriate nourishment is fundamental while participating in more extraordinary, even sporting physical exercise. Keeping up with energy balance is one of the fundamental assignments of satisfactory nourishment. Ideal nourishment gives energy to physical activity, works with recuperation from serious physical effort, and gives energy to invulnerable cells.

The utilization of starches increases with expanding force of activity (sugars oxidation raising), and simultaneously, the commitment of fat oxidation diminishes as the wellspring of energy.

Our body utilizes carbs more quickly than fat; in this manner, energy put away in sugars is all the more promptly accessible and utilizing rapidly. Eating food rich in carbs 2-3 hours before more extreme exercise to keep a high blood glucose level is suggested.

Thus, fats are a huge energy hotspot for moderate-force training. Nonetheless, physically dynamic individuals ought not have eaten less carbs wealthy in immersed fat. Proteins are a moderately minor wellspring of energy; however, they are significant for giving fundamental amino acids. We ought to consume them subsequent to working out. Lacking energy provided in food varieties impacts the invulnerable reaction to exceptionally escalated training.

Lacking supplements provided during dependable extreme focus training strengthens work out and incites safe melancholy. Carbs consumption during and after practice mitigates the unfriendly impacts of escalated practice on the resistant framework activity. Diet wealthy in starches diminishes the immunosuppressive impact of pressure chemicals.

Hydration is a basic part of our eating regimen that upholds our solid invulnerable framework. We ought to consume a fitting measure of liquids during activity and rest time to restrict the unsafe impacts of drying out on invulnerable capacities.

Keeping our skin and bodily fluid films all around hydrated is fundamental since they are the primary line of guard against infections and microbes. Water is likewise fundamental for lymph creation, a significant part of our guard framework.

Apparently, we as a whole realize that the nature of our rest is vital to our wellbeing and the working of the safe framework, so it merits putting in a couple of words on this point. Rest (and circadian cycle) considerably affects our immunological cycles.

Correspondence among apprehensive and safe frameworks is the premise of this impact intervened by different factors like synapses, cytokines, and chemicals. In addition, the autonomic sensory system straightforwardly innervates the resistant framework. The activity of the invulnerable framework is synchronized with our 24-hour rest wake cycle.

Unfortunate rest quality initiates a pressure reaction conjuring creation of favorable to incendiary cytokines, known as constant second rate irritation) and prompts immunodeficiency.

Ongoing rest interruption invigorates provocative cycles and may prompt expanded gamble of persistent infections like atherosclerosis, diabetes, rheumatoid joint inflammation, Crohn's illness, and disease.

Insufficient rest and low quality of rest increment the gamble of normal cold indications and work with different infections. Grown-ups who rest for under 7 hours daily have a multiple times higher gamble of fostering a typical cold and keeping up with their safe capacities in a decent state. Ideal rest term (7 to 8 hours) can help with the avoidance of cardiovascular illnesses or diabetes, for example.

The term physical activity covers an expansive range of our practices, frequently remembered for the class of wellbeing advancing practices. It is practically any sort of body development brought about by skeletal muscle withdrawals and influences each framework in our body.

We can say that a physically dynamic way of life is

a sort of return to our precursors' prior lifestyle in the time of hunting and assembling, millennia prior when physical wellness was a state of our endurance.

In current times our way of life is regularly excessively inactive, which is unnatural in our organic turn of events and can prompt physiological changes debilitating our safe framework and expanding our defenselessness to numerous illnesses.

Not all exercises or physical exercises are suitable for every one of us similarly. The first and most significant rule is to find those that will suit us and that will fulfill us, we will appreciate doing them.

For example, don't go to the rec center on the off chance that you lean toward outside exercises. Assuming you disdain running, just don't run and pick different exercises.

We can attempt different exercises prior to planning our activity plan; we can involve the Internet for this reason and consider whatever number choices as could be expected under the circumstances. The quantity of decisions accessible to browse is colossal, both inside and outside.

We have an enormous determination of aerobic exercises, obstruction training, strength training, and extreme cardio exercise while setting up our activity plan, posting the most well-known.

Aerobic exercises

This activity has numerous medical advantages. We can list the accompanying, expanding blood stream and internal heat level, lessening the quantity of harmful microorganisms, and assisting with keeping up with the right body weight by diminishing fat sum and to decrease aggravation; supporting our safe framework through moderate physical activity.

The motivation behind aerobic exercise is to work on the capacity of the heart and lungs to convey oxygen to create energy, which is vital for safe cell activity.

We as a rule recognize the accompanying sorts of exercises: cycling, running, swimming, and strolling. Every one of us can bring aerobic exercise into our day-by-day daily practice. Here are a few models:

climb the steps as opposed to utilizing lifts,

pick a vehicle leave found somewhat further from the spot of home or work,

ride a bike rather than a vehicle where conceivable,

strolling with your youngsters (close to the site of the home, for example).

Aerobic training rules could resemble this: recurrence 3 to 5 days per week, not more than 20 to 30 minutes every day in one meeting, or as a cumulative season of a few short meetings.

Opposition exercises

Opposition training works on our solid strength and power. The principal objective is to accomplish the most ideal capacity to apply a power and pressure at a given speed. Opposition training is tied in with making picked developments against any obstruction, for example, our body weight, utilizing chosen gear (free or machine loads), elastic groups, and others.

We should constantly remember the gamble of injury while playing out these exercises, particularly while utilizing high loads, unnecessary obstruction, or unseemly exercise strategies.

We should attempt to make the developments to their full scope of movement for each activity and never pause our breathing. The accompanying factors we ought to think about while arranging obstruction training: how much weight (assuming we use stacks), the quantity of redundancies, the speed of development, and the upkeep of muscle pressure.

We might build the force of our training by transforming one of the referenced elements. Two meetings each week are sufficient, and for every meeting, we should isolate by no less than two days off rest. We play out each activity by doing a limit of 12 reiterations, and we take a 2 brief break for rest.

Strength training

Building bulk is the fundamental justification behind doing strength exercises. Notwithstanding, we should bring up that they likewise have some significance for our resistant framework, chiefly in light of the fact that they are a storage facility of amino acids important for delivering antibodies and invulnerable cells like white platelets.

Fortunately, we can play out a critical piece of them at home without putting a truckload of cash in gym equipment; likewise, we don't need to utilize proficient exercise centers.

The instances of exercises that we can do at home are bouncing jacks, rushes, pullups, pushups, boards, or squats. We can present exercises with a free weight and a free weight to our arrangement of exercises. They add loads in normal exercises.

The most well-known free weight exercises are jumps and squats; we grasp a free weight before us or at our chest.

Flexibility training

We realize that flexibility decides the scope of movement in our joints. We ought to incorporate flexibility exercises in any training plans, particularly when more than 40 years of age, since they benefit physical capacities, and the scope of movement diminishes with age.

Ten minutes of flexibility (stretching) exercises performed 2-3 days of the week will be enough for keeping up with great flexibility in our joints. We should hold static stretches for 15-60 seconds (held movement with the end result of feeling inconvenience, not more).

Neuromuscular exercise

It is appropriate for more established grown-ups with a higher gamble of falling and they have utilitarian disabilities. We might incorporate Tai Chi, physical Yoga, and Pilates in our week after week training program and remember them for the gathering of neuromuscular training. We can consider neuromuscular training as a kind of flexibility training.

During the time spent arranging a bunch of exercises or our overall physical activity, we consider the accompanying parts: activity type, recurrence (how frequently seven days), span of every meeting, and force of each activity (for instance, weight, obstruction, speed of development).

Considering the wellbeing related parts, we talk about cardiorespiratory wellness, strong strength and perseverance, and flexibility. Practice span and recurrence have a reverse relationship with practice power.

We settle on decisions consistently whether or not we need to be all the more physically dynamic. Rather than driving via vehicle or transport, we can go for a stroll, climb steps as opposed to taking the lift, and walk a more extended distance than leaving close to the store or our home.

Whenever we need time, we can isolate our physical activity into more modest, a few minutes in length exercises played out a few times each day. For instance, somewhere around 10 minutes of training toward the beginning of the prior day breakfast and an additional 10 minutes around evening time prior to hitting the sack, and 10 to 20 minutes of a walk or moderate running during daytime.

We should take note of that inactive people would acquire critical advantages when they choose to be all the more physically dynamic and construct their own every day or week by week practice plans. We can incorporate extra wellbeing further developing exercises, for example, cycling, yard work, or moving at a sluggish speed.

Assume we need to move from a stationary way of life to being all the more physically dynamic. All things considered, we ought to aggregate our day-by-day activity as opposed to constraining ourselves to do extreme, comprehensive exercise, which can cause more damage than great for our wellbeing.

Everybody can practice at home

We have quite recently concluded that we should expand our physical activity to work on our wellbeing and prosperity. We need to decide if we will practice at home, in the exercise center, or outside in our closest area. Obviously, we can perform exercises utilizing straightforward gear, for example, hand weights, opposition belts, or home decorations.

Everything relies upon our demeanor, the space that we can dispense to the association of a little rec center for exercises, and, most importantly, on the monetary assets that we can spend on the acquisition of gear. We should always remember that we don't require specific gear to strengthen our resistant framework through physical activity.

Assuming that we choose to coordinate a small-scale rec center, we should figure out how exercises we will treat what hardware we should perform them. Prior to purchasing hardware for training, we should answer what our objective and kind of gear will be the most appropriate.

Will the picked hardware be really great for aerobic, strength, or flexibility training? For instance, in the event that we just arrange aerobic exercise outside our home, we don't require particular gear.

Allow us to check out the proposals given by American Council on Exercise (ACE), including the accompanying: how monetary assets treat need to spend on your home rec center, ensure hardware is customizable (for instance, would you be able to change it to your stature or the strength of your muscles).

Prior to purchasing any hardware, we should check whether we have an appropriate space for establishment or get together. For instance, for a fixed bike, we want 10 square feet (one square meter), free loads 20 to 60 square feet (2 to 5 square meters), treadmill 30 square feet (around 3 square meters), step stepper 10 to 20 square feet (1 to 2 square meters).

Assume we mean to utilize an exercise center or wellness focus. All things considered, we think about the accompanying: their area (pick an office close to home or work), take a gander at the expense (read the agreement cautiously), and search for an assortment of hardware and their condition.

Do the opening times match with our extra energy? Check for stopping, showers, bathrooms, storage spaces. Similarly significant is the request about the projects offered and the coaches.

Presently, a couple of words about outside physical activity. Undoubtedly, for some individuals, the indigenous habitat prompts both more youthful and more seasoned to be all the more physically dynamic and get additional joy from practicing in the outside air and a charming climate. The indigenous habitat, green spaces, specifically, influences some activity related factors like power and saw effort.

Metropolitan areas are exceptionally available for physical activity. Moreover, its vicinity to our place of home or work gives the extra advantage. Do you have any idea that youngsters are more dynamic in the neighborhood than at sports clubs, school, or home? Now and again our dread can be a serious deterrent to performing exercises close to our place of home or work.

At long last, some data on the dangers of physical activity. Do you have at least some ideas that the yearly rate for wounds ranges somewhere in the range of 37 and 56 percent among sporting sprinters? Lower appendage wounds are the most widely recognized, regularly brought about by consistent reiteration of a similar development (abuse, stress cracks), and just a small rate is unintentional falls.

Inclining factors remember absence of practicing

experience and fast increment for training power. Running on a hard surface and poor improper shoes are liable for close to 5 percent of wounds.

Low to direct power physical activity (strolling, for instance) doesn't make any gamble of outer muscle wounds and our wellbeing. Too escalated effort can build the gamble of cardiovascular failure, which is a serious issue for individuals with existing heart sickness. We ought to constantly change the training plan for our wellbeing and physical capacities.

CHAPTER 3
AEROBIC TRAINING TO
INCREASE RESISTANCE.

Aerobics, which in a real sense implies with oxygen, are practices that should be possible to get thinner and recover wellbeing. There are primary kinds of aerobic exercises, and assuming you do these exercises day by day, you will see that you truly will be sounder. Aerobics are by and large done at moderate degrees of force for a more drawn-out time frame and can focus on any piece of your body you wish to thin. There are many benefits of aerobics, which is the reason this type of activity is both significant and well known among wellbeing cognizant individuals.

Exercise can be separated into two classifications: aerobic and anaerobic. These contrast in the ways in which your muscles contract during the activity and how energy is created inside the muscles. Instances of anaerobic exercises incorporate weight training or strength training, and with aerobic exercises, even the most fabricated jock cannot run, swim, and so on for significant stretches of time.

During aerobic exercise, your body separates glycogen to use for energy. In the event that there isn't sufficient glycogen in the body, you begin utilizing fat stores all things considered, which is the reason you get thinner. Oxygen assumes a critical part in this cycle. With aerobic exercise, you don't use explosions of energy. Rather, you spread out moderate degrees of energy throughout an extensive stretch of time to set off the utilization of fat in energy creation. As a rule, things like running significant distances, aerobics moves, and swimming for extensive stretches of time are viewed as aerobics exercises, while anything with short eruptions of movement, such as running, are not.

Advantages of aerobics exercises are incredible, which is the reason most specialists prescribe them to patients, regardless of whether you partake in a typical weight. A portion of these advantages incorporate strengthening the repertory muscles, expanding the heart to siphon all the more productively, expanding the progression of blood (and oxygen) in the body, and expanding perseverance. Aerobics decline the gamble of death because of cardiovascular issues and of osteoporosis in all kinds of people.

Need to figure out how aerobics can transform you? There are various incredible exercise programs you can do, which incorporate both independent exercises and classes with gatherings. To find out additional (and consistently prior to beginning another practicing program, converse with your primary care physician or other medical services proficient to realize what sorts of aerobic exercises will turn out best for your body. Aerobics are the way to living a better and physically useful life, so don't stand by one more day prior to beginning another sound program that incorporates aerobics.

Aerobics for Beginners

Assuming that you are simply beginning with aerobics, you may be feeling overpowered. The facts confirm that there are numerous ways of working out, and that assuming you can figure out how to get a decent workout you will be a lot better. It is additionally a fact that you really want to have a course of workout wherein your body is moving quickly and your heart and lungs are compelled to work more earnestly than when you are very still. This is called aerobic exercise, and it is something vital that you comprehend.

Don't believe that you need to begin at the upper immediately. Progressed aerobics can be something that you need to work up to. This remembers running for place and doing a progression of developments that you could see as exceptionally threatening to begin with. And furthermore, it isn't protected to begin anyplace other than as an amateur, since you could hurt yourself and you likewise could run into issues. In this manner, you need to begin all along to have the option to get the most advantage from your daily schedule.

Starting aerobics are exceptionally simple and they are something that you can do even from home. The point is to get your blood streaming, so starting aerobics involves starting with strolling set up and moving your arms and legs to get your pulse up. Then, at that point, you steadily continue to accomplish an ever-increasing number of developments and to do them quicker.

Something extraordinary to accomplish for starting aerobics is to begin by strolling or running set up. You can then fire moving your arms all over. The mark of aerobics is to get your heart rolling, and the most effective way to do this is to continue to do developments, such as bouncing jacks, for however many redundancies as you can do. This is the most ideal way for you to begin with aerobic training, since you can move gradually up from nothing and truly get looking great as you do this.

Something different that you should remember is that aerobics regularly work better to music. The way that it works is that you can utilize the music to keep your rhythm and to keep your buckling down. You can likewise time your exercises to music - you can do one set for a whole melody, for example. Music can be your inspiration and it can assist you with continuing to work out.

Aerobic Exercise, No Matter What Your Age

Everybody needs to get better, and everybody knows what all things considered, doing aerobic exercise consistently is something that can truly take you from a reason behind being undesirable, and carry you to a spot where you can be solid and you can partake in all that life brings to the table for you. This goes for everybody, except there are sure gatherings who need to plan their aerobic exercise cautiously to try not to hurt themselves.

Seniors are in one of these gatherings. With regards to aerobic exercise for seniors, there are a few things that you need to consider before you start. Recollect that for everybody, aerobic exercise is something that you will need to move toward. You should begin little, and where you start will rely a great deal upon the fact that you are so beneficial to start with. To get better, you need to go from where you are and work up. This goes for seniors also.

Seniors must take stock of all of their wellbeing before they start to have aerobic exercise consistently. This is on the grounds that seniors are more inclined to medical issues as a general rule, so they should see their PCP before they start doing aerobic exercise and they ought to counsel a specialist prior to rolling out any significant improvements to the way that they get work out.

Notwithstanding, after they have seen a specialist, seniors can start a regiment of aerobic exercise in only the equivalent way as individuals of all ages. Except if their PCP has recommended that they don't do aerobics for reasons unknown, a senior should start with a short workout, and steadily move gradually up to longer exercises. This is the same way that others should begin an aerobic exercise program. Assuming seniors adhere to these guidelines, and in the event that they do nothing that they feel their body can't deal with, they ought to have similar outcomes with aerobic exercise as any other individual.

Everything relies upon the fact that you are so beneficial to start with, and how far you need to take the activity. However long you don't get carried away, an aerobics workout will be exceptionally useful for you.

Recall however, similar to any other individual, you ought to talk about your arrangements with your PCP, regardless of whether you feel that you are totally sound. Your primary care physician will have more data regarding what kind of activity will be best for you.

Aerobics are extremely helpful types of activity, regardless of the region of your body you are attempting to focus for weight reduction. They should likewise be possible just to partake in a better life. Aerobics have the additional advantage of assisting members with building perseverance too. Subsequently, there truly is not a great explanation for the vast majority to not do aerobics! Nonetheless, before you start any sort of new medical care schedule, it is critical to figure out how precisely aerobics work. You can do this in various ways.

As a matter of first importance, you want to converse with your PCP to settle on the most ideal wellbeing choices. A specialist will actually want to reject aerobics programs that won't be gainful for your body, appear to be excessively challenging for your ability level, or really could cause injury. A specialist can likewise disclose to you the best aerobic exercises to do during your daily schedule, suggest mentors, and disclose to you all of the extraordinary medical advantages of aerobics-and accept me, there are loads of them. Your first stop ought to consequently be your PCP's office. Ensure that you pass on sufficient time during the arrangement to pose bunches of inquiries that you might have.

The Internet is additionally an incredible asset with regards to tracking down data on aerobics. Not exclusively would you be able to peruse articles about the advantages and history of aerobics, yet you can interface in talk rooms and discussions with others to share aerobics encounters and pose inquiries. The Internet likewise allows you to check out explicit schedules and a few sites even assist you with assembling aerobics designs that work for you!

Past the Internet, you can likewise get more familiar with aerobics utilizing customary writing regarding the matter. Your nearby library ought to have an assortment of books that you can peruse, and assuming you see that the assets there are excessively obsolete, you can likewise glance around at the closest book shop. Assuming you track down books that you like, you might have the option to buy them at limited costs online in various spots.

Wellness magazines are important too. While the data on the Internet may not be composed by experts, articles you'll find in magazines have as a rule been checked for realities and altered by various individuals in the medical services field. Finding out with regards to aerobics is easy. Since individuals are starting to feel more wellbeing cognizant, this kind of data is currently surrounding us.

Aerobics to Target the Abdomen

We as a whole realize that working out is something vital for us to do. You will need to get a workout so you can be better, thus that you know how you are treating it comes to improving point of view. The vast majority of individuals who get discouraged and undesirable aren't doing aerobics, so regardless of your degree of wellbeing, aerobics will be great for you.

Be that as it may, now and then it is critical to target more than one region with regards to aerobics. You should deal with something specifically. Regularly, individuals have portions of their bodies that they don't like however much that others do, and this can be exceptionally unpleasant. More often than not, workouts try to make your entire body more grounded, and keeping in mind that this is significant, assuming you have a trouble spot, you could feel like you need to work it out.

To focus on the mid-region while you are doing aerobics, you actually must recollect what the mid-region is and why it is significant. It isn't simply your belly region; this is an entire scope of muscles that help you move and stretch in each piece of your day-by-day daily schedule. This is the reason focusing on your midsection during aerobics is vital.

Whenever you are checking out focusing on your midsection, consider first redundancies. The most ideal way to chip away at your mid-region is to add stretches into anything you are doing aerobically. In the event that you are strolling or running, you ought to extend your body and stretch from one side to another as you move. You must be certain that the development you are making is coming to structure your mid-region, notwithstanding. It is all around simple to move your arms and legs and think that you are stretching your midsection.

Another extraordinary thing that you can do while you are doing your aerobics is to stoop down and to then utilize your midsection muscles to go all over into various positions. Recollect that you need to continue to do reiterations at a sufficiently high pace to keep your pulse up. The more that you move, the better in shape you will get. This is an incredible method for focusing on your midsection. Again, however ensure that the developments are coming from your belly region.

Aerobics from your Living Room: Working Out at Home

There are numerous ways that you can make aerobics work for you. Above all else, you should see how indispensable aerobic workouts are to your wellbeing. You can get solid just by strolling and by lifting loads, yet to be really sound, you need to figure out how to get your heart pumping and to get your blood streaming. To this end aerobic exercise is the most critical to you; it truly permits you to get every one of the pieces of your body cooperating. Consequently, everybody sees how significant aerobic workouts can be.

Be that as it may, now and again you essentially can't go to the rec center or take a class to get better and to have better aerobic workouts. Many individuals are occupied with family and with work responsibilities, and going to a rec center or class just doesn't meet their requirements. There must be something that individuals can do at home for their aerobic workout, correct?

There are numerous things, indeed, that you can do to do aerobics at home. The essential basics of aerobic workouts incorporate the way that you need to get your heart pumping and your breathing rate up. These things can be achieved in numerous ways.

Assuming you are keen on aerobics at home, you

should realize that there are a few things you can do to achieve this. Above all else, the most famous way of doing your aerobic workout at home is to get a bicycle or a treadmill. This is the sort of thing that you can have in an advantageous spot in your home and it tends to be prepared for you at whatever point you have the opportunity and willpower to work out. Both of these are incredible ways of ensuring that you get your aerobic workout.

Another extraordinary thing that you can do is foster a daily schedule for yourself at home that remembers running for place, working out with rope, or in any event, going around your area or somewhere near you. These things are vital in light of the fact that you can alter your workout to meet your requirements, and this can be an incredible method for getting in shape. To work out, yet you have had the opportunity and energy to go to a class or to join an exercise center, this can be the best and ideal opportunity for you to snag something like a bicycle, a treadmill, or a running schedule that you can do from home.

Well known Aerobics Machines

With regards to aerobics, you could observe that you improve your workout on a machine rather than really running or hopping rope. Recollect that like all aspects of a sound workout schedule, aerobics are exercises that must be customized to your body and what is best for your wellbeing. You need to cooperate with your primary care physician and your fitness coach assuming you have one to foster a framework for working out that works for you, and to ensure that anything you are doing is awesome for your body and your brain too.

Machines have become exceptionally well known with regards to working out on the grounds that occasionally they are simpler to utilize and more straightforward to become acclimated to. You don't need to stress over running outside when it is cold out or figuring out how to get your workout when you don't have time assuming you have a machine in your home that you can utilize.

CHAPTER 4

THE BENEFITS OF AEROBIC TRAINING FOR THE HEART IN PEOPLE OVER 60.

There are more advantages of aerobics for your body that you might actually count. All around this present reality, individuals are discussing new and better ways of working out, on the grounds that all around the world the well-being of individuals is falling into extremely hazardous regions. That implies that specialists and other medical care experts have been discussing the advantages of aerobics for quite a while. You also can take advantage of this get sort of activity.

There are essentially an excessive number of advantages of aerobics to make reference to rapidly. Notwithstanding, there are not many that stick out as vital. For example, the most ideal way that you can ensure you are carrying on with a sound life is to get your pulse siphoning, and the very best method for getting your pulse going is to find something that you can do like aerobics, that requires steady development with practically no resting in request to be genuinely solid, you must have the option to have a consistent development and to get your pulse going for a time span. Permitting your heart to continue going at a higher rate than resting temporarily is probably the most ideal way to get sound, since this conveys blood and oxygen to each piece of your body at a much quicker rate.

There are likewise a lot more advantages of aerobics that you probably won't have even understood. Other than making your heart and lungs solid, aerobics makes each of your muscles more grounded in light of the fact that you need to keep them moving for longer time frames ceaselessly. This implies that regardless of the piece of your body you are focusing your aerobics on working, you will observe that you are getting increasingly strong over the long haul.

You should converse with a specialist assuming you are keen on getting a full rundown of the advantages of aerobics, yet realize immediately that there are a large number. Before you start an aerobics schedule, in any case, you should be certain that you are conversing with your primary care physician, since there are certain individuals who need to move gradually up to a full-fledged routine in view of other medical problems. Be certain that you have the go-ahead from your primary care physician so you can begin on getting the advantages of aerobics directly to yourself! You won't ever feel so particularly great as when you are working out and dealing with yourself, and getting into an aerobics routine is the most ideal way for you to achieve this.

Advantages of a Personal Trainer for Aerobic Exercise

There are ordinarily in your life that you should have the assistance of a fitness coach, and doing aerobic exercise is absolutely one of those times. This is what is going on in which a fitness coach can truly assist you with benefiting from your wellness objectives and can truly assist you with sorting out where you should go next with regards to working out.

It is extremely simple to track down a mentor to assist you with your aerobic exercise. Interestingly, you can observe a mentor that comprehends what your identity is and can assist you with being all that you can be. There are many sorts of coaches that could fit this thought, so you must be certain that you observe one that truly causes you to feel good. It could appear as though a mentor that worries you would be really great for your working out, yet over the long haul you could wind up getting more baffled and you probably won't wind up doing as well as you might want to do.

The purpose in having a fitness coach is that you are truly permitted to act naturally and to do everything that you can manage all alone. This implies that you must work with the guidance of a coach, however all things considered you must have the option to deal with yourself and improve shape. Your individual coach should be somebody who will energize you yet in addition somebody who will allow you to act naturally and work at your own speed.

Whenever you have a fitness coach for aerobic exercise, you can rely on one thing you will have inspiration. Regularly, aerobic exercise is something simple to disregard and something simple to place as a second thought due to different things that surface. With your fitness coach you'll observe that it is a lot harder to escape working, so you will be bound to finish your workout. However long you can observe a fitness coach that will work with you and that will work with any circumstances that you could have; you will see that this can be generally gainful for yourself and you'll have the option to be extremely cheerful with regards to how much work that you have done.

CHAPTER 5
STRENGTH TRAINING TO
IMPROVE MUSCLE FLEXIBILITY.

Tragically as we age, we lose muscle, which might prompt sensations of delicacy and loss of autonomy. Notwithstanding, it doesn't need to be like this: there are a few things you can do to battle the impacts of maturing and develop your fortitude so you feel fitter and surer. Perhaps the most effective way to do this is by taking part in strength training.

Strength training includes utilizing opposition, (for example, weight machines or rec center packs) to build muscle size and power. It is not the same as intense exercise, which develops your cardiovascular framework.

Core standards of strength training exercise

The expression "center rule" is characterized as "(in sport) the basic thought or message that something represents." Many individuals accept that one of the center standards in strength training exercises is to guarantee maximal power creation.

The standards underneath are the essentials of strength training for all levels, from amateurs to cutting edge competitors.

Structure should be right: The execution of each activity ought to stress the right structure and method. This includes utilizing appropriate body mechanics during the developments.

Fluctuated Intensity: Ensure that your workout routine incorporates low, moderate and focused energy units all through the month to keep your muscles tested and forestall transformation. These units need not be progressive inside a given week as they are disseminated over time.

Assortment: As you progress through your training cycle, you should change your exercises. The body adjusts explicitly to the forced requests, so proceeding with progress is just conceivable assuming the body is constantly tested with more prominent over-burdens.

Movement: Ensure that you are step by step expanding the opposition for each activity over the long run as this is one more significant boost expected for progress.

Rest and Recovery: Strength is worked during recuperation, not in the middle of sets. Plan to plan a few rest days of the week.

Keep Reps Low: Decreasing rep range by 1 rep for each set can be an incredible method for expanding the power and receive every one of the rewards of strength training.

Recurrence: To advance outcomes, strength training ought to be performed 2-3 times each week.

Center: The psyche and body association is indispensable for strength training. Keep up with the center during each set and envision your muscles working all through the scope of movement. This will cause the activity to appear to be simpler, which initiates less muscle strands, permitting you to play out a more noteworthy number of reps with a given weight load.

Compound Movements: Exercises, for example, squats, seat press, shoulder press, and pull-ups work for a long-time muscle bunch at the same time, so they are viewed as compound exercises. These exercises require huge energy, so it is ideal to perform them before separation or machine-based exercises that target individual muscle bunches on exchanging days.

Movement: Ensure that you are step by step expanding the opposition for each activity after some time, as this is one more significant upgrade expected for progress. Section level exercisers should mean to build reps and burden, though transitional and progressed competitors should zero in on keeping a steady rep range while advancing burden from multi week to another. It is imperative to recall that dynamic over-burden is the boost for proceeding with progress in all cases.

Reiteration Speed: To target explicit muscle filaments inside a given muscle bunch, you should play out certain lifts dangerously (whimsical stage) and different lifts all the more intentionally (concentric stage).

Why Strength Training

Strength training for seniors is an incredible method for keeping the body and psyche dynamic and sound. A great many people start strength training in their late adolescents or mid-twenties since they see the fastest muscle development, yet ongoing exploration shows that significantly more established grown-ups can profit from ordinary obstruction workouts.

The way to forestall sarcopenia (muscle misfortune) is moderate over-burden (steadily expanding every year). This implies beginning sluggishness and advancing gradually while remembering security. A compelling system ought to incorporate 8-10 exercises for every meeting focusing on all significant muscle gatherings, including quads, hamstrings, hip adductors, hip abductors, glutes, lats, biceps/rear arm muscles, shoulders/center, and calves/abs.

Each activity ought to be performed for two arrangements of 10-15 reps with something like brief reprieve in the middle of sets.

Strength training will build bulk, which has been displayed to diminish by and large body weight (because of diminished fat mass) and further develop rest quality, decreasing the gamble of injury, diabetes, osteoporosis, coronary illness, dementia, and sorrow.

In addition, since strength is relative (strength can differ contingent upon age), seniors may at first neutralize lighter protections until they become acclimated to physically burdening exercises like obstruction training.

Strength training information

Strength training information is very useful for all individuals, particularly the older. Regardless of whether you are not extremely impressive, you can in any case work on your wellbeing and forestall delicacy via training in strength. Strength training isn't just about building up like a muscle head; basically, one more type of activity can assist you with getting more grounded and be more adaptable. Each kind of activity has its advantages, which is the reason you ought to consider strength training as well.

There are numerous physiological motivations to take up weight training. One of the most significant is that it discharges development chemicals to fabricate bone and bulk. This can assist with forestalling a few infections like osteoporosis and joint pain as well. For instance, assuming you have frail muscles, the bones will become more vulnerable. Along these lines, being solid can assist your body with remaining sound and shield you from certain infections.

One more motivation to lift loads is that it builds your metabolic rate. Not exclusively will you consume more calories when you are working out, however for a really long time later. Weight training forestalls age-related muscle misfortune, making exercises like climbing steps and conveying regular food items harder further down the road. This is particularly significant for seniors since an unfortunate stance or balance can break.

Getting started

For the individuals who haven't been occupied with much physical activity in some time, it might very well be insightful to talk with a specialist prior to starting.

Beginning with strength and power training relies upon the exercises you select.

Utilizing hand weights or strength-training machines is a choice and depends exclusively on your body weight. Certain individuals like to work out in a rec center, while others work out at home. There are a couple of things that impact strength training you really want to know before you start.

Everyone is unique

Practicing doesn't need to be done similarly for everybody. It is conceivable that two people doing a likewise training system can accomplish immensely various outcomes. For a really long time, one individual would invest the energy at the exercise center, yet their training accomplice is getting more grounded each time.

What labors for a 60-year-close buddy may not work for you, so it's memorable and vital that everybody's body frameworks are unique.

Sex

Ladies' cooperation in sports was once viewed as

unseemly and inadmissible, however these contentions have been dismissed, and ladies currently take an interest in most donning exercises. In some ultra-perseverance occasions, ladies are viewed as better than men, and the hole among people's achievements is restricting.

Hereditary make-up

All parts of wellness and execution, including muscle and strength, are impacted by one's hereditary qualities. Somewhat, qualities impact our capacities, from runners with all the quicker jerk muscle fiber to perseverance sprinters whose qualities direct muscle withdrawal speeds.

Numerous qualities are associated with muscle development and advancement. Researchers have found numerous qualities associated with muscle development. It's hazy the way in which they're included, yet it is exceptionally difficult. Furthermore, more muscle-developing qualities are relied upon to be found later on.

Social-social foundation

Individuals' interest in physical activity is impacted by different social and individual elements, including their age, orientation, nationality, and handicap.

Competitors of any age, sexual orientations, races, religions, and societies partake in sports.

Age

Injury recuperation time increments as an individual's physical wellness lessens as they progress in years. Golf, bowls, and cycling are well known with the old since they are less difficult and require less physical effort.

Nationality

In certain networks, nationality, and orientation consolidate to greatly affect interest than they would alone. The level of South Asian physically dynamic ladies is 92%, contrasted with 55% of all ladies.

Practice Myths

Practice is great all the time. It keeps the joints greased up, forms muscle and strengthens bones, further develops balance and coordination, hones center, lessens pressure and sorrow, builds endurance, so you feel more grounded each day... Yet, imagine a scenario where it's past the point of no return. Imagine a scenario where you have been carrying on with an inactive life for quite a long time. Is there actually a desire to start an activity program at age 60 or over? Obviously, there is!

Exercise will kill me! It will make me feel like the other elderly folks.

Advantages of activity for seniors

As individuals age, they should manage a few physical difficulties that make day by day undertakings more troublesome. With customary exercise, seniors can work on their balance and muscle strength to upgrade portability. Likewise, senior residents might look over aerobic exercises pointed toward further developing heart wellbeing or weight-bearing exercises intended to slow bone misfortune and forestall osteoporosis.

Further develop state of mind and emotional wellness

While it is generally expected information among wellness mentors that activity can help one's physical wellbeing, researchers currently broadly acknowledge that the benefits stretch out a long way past the physical casing. The human body goes through many changes as an individual ages, in the actual body as well as in the psyche.

CHAPTER 6

BALANCE TRAINING TO

PREVENT FALLS.

How does our body keep up with balance and harmony? There are three principal body frameworks that add to our general balance. These incorporate tangible contributions from three regions of our bodies, the handling of that information, and our bodies response to the information.

Tactile Input

Our minds get data from all pieces of our bodies. For balance, the mind especially takes a gander at the nerve motivations received from the eyes, the ears, and the muscles and joints in our arms and legs.

• Visual. The bars and cones in our eyes send messages to the mind to assist it with figuring out where our bodies are according to our environmental elements. These viewable prompts assist us with drawing closer or stay away from things in our way and keep us adjusted.

- Contact. Sensors in our skin, muscles, and joints hand-off data with the goal that our cerebrum knows when we are moving forward, what direction our head is turned, and where our body is in the space we are possessing.

- Vestibular. The internal trenches and working of our ears make up most of the vestibular framework. It adds to the consciousness of harmony and movement. The driving forces that the sensors ship off the cerebrum permits us to know whether we are standing, resting, or turning, in addition to other things.

Mix of Input

The approach together of all the information got in the mind is separated and appointed to specific pieces of the cerebrum. The cerebrum stem joins and sorts data from the faculties.

- Cerebellum. Called the coordination focus of the mind, the cerebellum controls stance and balance. It depends on programmed responses and past history from rehashed openness to specific activities. This is the piece of the cerebrum that assists a racquetball player with realizing what sort of balance they should serve the ball.

• Cerebral cortex. This reasoning and memory war room of the cerebrum adds to memory and decisive reasoning, similar to independent direction. Putting away data in this space assists an individual with recollecting that strolling on a stormy road requires additional alert due to slip dangers and smooth surfaces.

Engine Input

At last, the cerebrum stem again comes into the image. It sends messages to all regions of the body and instructs it to keep up with balance. A few reflexes include:

• Eye reflex. Called the vestibulo-visual reflex, this programmed capacity of our eyes is set off by the data coming from the cerebrum. It permits your look to stay consistent, regardless of whether your head is moving from one side to another or all over.

• Engine motivations. These regulate eye developments and make body changes. With the data from the mind, your muscles and joints can move in the manner they need to in light of data from your eyes. Assuming you have at any point seen an artist or ice skater whirl around and around over and over while keeping their balance, you have seen this engine motivation in real life.

Feeling of dread toward Falling

Marilyn was a mother and grandma who wanted to invest energy with her children and grandkids consistently. She wanted to heat with her grandchildren and take them to the motion pictures. At one time, Marilyn was an enthusiastic tennis player, but since she was presently in her mid-seventies, she didn't play as much tennis as she used to. She likewise didn't want to go to the rec center any longer in light of the fact that the activity classes were simply excessively hard for her. Her joints turned out to be creakier and her joint inflammation erupted occasionally, yet generally she was doing affirm. She was in the kitchen one day, going after a baking dish that was at the rear of the rack, when she lost her balance and fell. As she was falling, she hit her head on the edge of the ledge prior to arriving on her hip on the kitchen tile flooring. She ended up with a joint for the cut on her temple and a messed-up hip that expected a medical procedure. On account of the wounds she sustained, Marilyn lost her versatility, yet lost a portion of her autonomy to drive and get around all alone also.

Falls are not a typical piece of maturing. However, consistently, a huge number of more seasoned grown-ups lose their balance, fall, and harm themselves. The Center for Disease Control (CDC) measurements connected with falls are calming. They include:

• One-fourth of grown-ups north of 65 years of age fall every year.

• When you fall, your opportunity for falling again pairs.

• Trauma centers the country over see north of 3,000,000 more seasoned grown-ups for wounds connected with falls and 800,000 of those are hospitalized in light of head or hip wounds that are an outcome from their fall.

- One-fifth of falls cause genuine injury like head injury or broken bones.

- Horrible cerebrum wounds are generally ordinarily brought about by a fall.

- North of 95% of hip cracks are the aftereffect of a fall (CDC, 2019).

While falls may not consistently cause genuine injury, a fifth of the time, the wounds are terrible enough that it becomes hard for the harmed individual to achieve regular exercises, drive, or live freely.

Fall Risk Factors

While anybody can unintentionally excursion and fall, there are sure circumstances that make it more probable for you to fall. These gamble factors include:

- Vision issues. As a result, old enough and either injury or ailment, we can encounter issues with our vision. Not having the option to see objects at our feet or in our pathway can make us stagger over them and possibly fall.

• Foot torment. Having foot torment can happen from one or the other injury to the foot or just from sick fitting shoes that need backing and hold. To keep up with balance, we really want the tangible criticism from our feet, lower legs, knees, and hips.

• Remedy and over-the-counter drugs. Specialist recommended drugs can in some cases cause discombobulation or tiredness, particularly torment prescription, narcotics, sedatives, and antidepressants. OTC drugs like allergy meds, hack syrups, and cold meds can likewise influence your consistent quality on your feet.

• Lack of vitamin D. The connection between vitamin D and great bone wellbeing is grounded. There is likewise some proof that when vitamin D levels fall under a specific point in the body, muscle working is diminished and the gamble for falls expands (Akdeniz et al., 2016).

• Trip risks in the home. Lopsided advances, free covering or floor tiles, electrical ropes, and area rugs are largely normal excursion perils at home. Poor or faint lighting, things left on the floor, and water or other fluid that has spilled on the floor are different perils that can add to falls.

• Center and lower body shortcoming. More established grown-ups can once in a while become unfortunate of falling and scale back their physical exercises. Sadly, the familiar axiom "in the event that you don't utilize it, you lose it" is valid with regards to center and leg strength. Less endurance and strength in the lower half of the body is a contributing variable in the event of falls.

Four Ways to Prevent Falls

Since we realize what can add to falls as we become older, we will investigate how we can be proactive and keep tumbles from occurring. Keep in mind, falling is anything but a typical piece of maturing! It is avoidable with only a couple of preplanned steps, for example,

• Have your eyes and feet analyzed. The specialist won't just glance at the general wellbeing of your vision, however can recommend a refreshed remedy for glasses or contacts also. Clear vision is important to stay away from falls. Have your medical services supplier take a gander at your feet and the shoes you ordinarily wear, and get a proposal for a podiatrist if essential.

•   Get a yearly exam. Consistently, get an appraisal of your wellbeing from your overall expert or medical care supplier. Consult with your primary care physician about any tipsiness or balance that you have had and have them audit the rundown of professionally prescribed prescriptions you take to check whether there are any connections that might add to sensations of dazedness, sleepiness, or unsteadiness. Get some information about vitamin D enhancements that can work on your bone and muscle wellbeing.

•   Make your home excursion resistant. Clean all the strolling region of your home off of any messiness, books, or little articles that you might conceivably fall over. Eliminate disperse mats or tape them down safely with twofold sided floor covering tape. Use non-slip mats in the restroom and different regions that have tile flooring. Keep generally involved things in simple to-arrive at spots to try not to utilize step stools or stepping stools. Evaluate the lighting in your home and change out lights or bulbs for ones that proposition clear, warm lights to assist you with seeing better.

• Keep a normal work out regime. Talk about with your PCP or a physical coach how you can practice securely and fuse cardiovascular, strength training, adaptability, and balance exercises into an everyday schedule. As you gain strength, endurance, and certainty, you decline your possibilities of falling and hurting yourself.

Test Your Balance

How great is your balance? Whenever we are youthful, our balance and response times are normally great. As we age, in any case, things happen that influence our strength like disease, injury, and ailments. Balance is pivotal to performing regular exercises and keeping away from falls, and it is not difficult to test our balance at home to find out about how we are doing.

Something imperative to recall prior to testing out your balance all alone is to be straightforward with yourself and the current state of your wellbeing. It is typical to feel dazed and cockeyed in the event that you are sick, affected by liquor or certain prescriptions, or tired. Be that as it may, assuming you are encountering persistent dizziness and balance issues, you should see a specialist to have things looked at. A few admonition signs that mean it's an ideal opportunity to look for clinical assessment include:

•   Intermittent episodes of unsteadiness for reasons unknown.

•   Discombobulation that goes on for more than a few days.

•   Ongoing tipsiness that outcomes in the failure to walk or drive securely.

•   Tipsiness that happens after a fall or mishap.

•   Indications of disarray, slurred discourse, shortcoming, or deadness on one side of the body.

Types of exercises

In reverse Walking

Length of activity: 30 seconds

Absolute time: 3 minutes

Regions chipped away at: abs, glutes, hips, quadriceps, hamstrings, calves, lower legs

Headings:

This activity is best finished with an accomplice that can make you aware of any stumbling risks. Make certain to stroll on a level, level region. Assuming you are on a walkway, ensure you are away from traffic and different people on foot. This should likewise be possible on a treadmill.

To begin, stroll forward 10 stages. Pivot and keep on strolling in a similar heading yet confronting in reverse. Walk gradually for 10 stages. Pivot again and keep on strolling 10 stages forward.

Rehash for 2 minutes, switching back and forth between strolling 10 stages looking ahead and 10 stages confronting in reverse all while strolling in one heading.

To step up: Once you are happy with strolling in reverse, stroll for 20 stages rather than 10 stages.

Observe: This activity helps your center muscles

react to directional changes as well as working your leg muscles in various ways. Go for care not to stroll excessively fast while strolling in reverse to abstain from falling.

Balance Walking

Length of activity: brief 30 seconds

Complete time: 3 minutes

Regions chipped away at: shoulders, abs, hip flexors, glutes, hamstrings, lower legs

Headings:

Standing up tall, bring your arms up and out directly from the sides of your body to about bear stature.

Move forward with your right foot and as you bring your left foot from behind you to make the following stride, twist your left knee and lift your left foot up. Stop for 1 second prior to finishing the remainder of the progression forward with your left foot.

Do exactly the same thing now with your right foot. As you present your right leg for the subsequent stage, twist your right knee and lift the right foot, holding it up for 1 second prior to finishing the progression. Rehash for 20 stages.

Yet again rest for a couple of moments, then, at that point, rehash work out.

Observe: This activity is like the standing walks yet with positive progress. The lower leg muscles are being strengthened as they assist your body with settling. Assuming you want support, have an accomplice hold one of your hands.

Ball Toss

Length of activity: 30 seconds

All out time: brief 30 seconds

Regions dealt with: hands, lower arms, glutes, hip flexors, hamstrings, calves

Bearings:

Carry a little soft ball with you on your walk. As you stroll forward, crush the ball in your right hand as you walk 10 stages forward.

Throw the ball to your left hand and crush the ball in

your left hand as you keep strolling for another 10 stages.

Rehash two additional times in each hand.

Observe: By having to perform various tasks, your body will change its balance and coordination. Be certain you keep your eyes zeroed in on where you are strolling to abstain from stumbling.

Check Walking

Length of activity: 30 seconds

Absolute time: 30 seconds

Regions dealt with: abs, hips, glutes, internal thighs, hamstrings, calves

Headings:

Have a go at strolling in an orderly fashion on a somewhat raised surface like a two-by-four length of wood or a check. Assuming you are outside, be certain that you are heading some place in the opposite direction from traffic and with a companion. You can put your hand on their shoulder for help or hold their arm.

On the off chance that you are uncertain with regards to strolling on something as tall as a control, take a stab at strolling in an orderly fashion, heel-to-toe, on a level way.

Observe: This activity requires a smaller position, which provides you with a more modest base of security. Walk slow and heel-to-toe to try not to tumble off the check.

Dynamic Walking

Length of activity: 30 seconds

All out time: 5 minutes

Regions dealt with: neck, abs, hip flexors, glutes, hamstrings, calves

Bearings:

Do this first in your lounge or lawn until you become acclimated to it. Beginning toward one side of your room or yard, walk gradually towards the contrary side.

While proceeding to walk straight, gradually turn your head to the right and afterward to the left while strolling. Keep turning your head to the right and left

98

leisurely until you arrive at the opposite side of the room.

Rehash multiple times.

To step up: As you get more certain, you can join this into your strolls outside at the recreation area or in your area.

Observe: This activity requires a change in your concentrate each time you turn your head. Make certain to turn your head gradually to keep away from unsteadiness. Assuming you feel dazed whenever, stop.

Grapevine

Length of activity: 1 minutes

Absolute time: 5 minutes

Regions chipped away at: abs, hips, internal thighs, quadriceps, calves

Headings:

You can clutch a ledge as you do this activity or have an accomplice clutch your hands in the event that you feel flimsy.

Begin by standing up tall with your feet together. Get your right foot over your left and step down. Uncross by bringing your left foot back and putting it close on your right side so the two feet are together regularly. Keep getting your right foot over your left for 10 stages or until you arrive at the opposite finish of the ledge.

Head back in the other path at this point crossing your left foot behind your right and venturing to the right. Uncross by bringing your right foot up and setting it close on your left side. Keep crossing your abandoned foot as you travel to one side for 10 stages or arrive at the finish of the counter.

Rehash multiple times.

To step up: If you become extremely familiar with this activity, you can make it more testing by rotating crossing in front and intersection behind each and every other advance.

Observe: At first you might end up peering down at your feet, however make sure to gaze upward and see where you are going. Attempt to keep your head up.

Heel-to-Toe

Length of activity: 30 seconds

Absolute time: 2 minutes 30 seconds

Regions chipped away at: abs, hips, internal thighs, quadriceps, hamstrings, calves

Bearings:

You can clutch a ledge as you do this activity or have an accomplice clutch your hands assuming you feel precarious.

Stand up tall and put your right foot straightforwardly before your left. Walk heel-to-toe as though you were strolling on a tightrope. Keep strolling heel-to-toe for 15 stages or until you arrive at the opposite finish of the counter or inverse side of the room.

Rehash multiple times.

To step up: To make this seriously difficult, you can put veiling tape or blue painters' tape in an orderly fashion on your floor. Work on strolling on the line, without clutching anything.

Observe: This activity requires a smaller position and will challenge your balance due to a more modest base of help. You can raise your arms from your sides to assist with solidness in the event that you are not clutching anything.

Avoids

Length of activity: 45 seconds

Complete time: 4 minutes

Regions chipped away at: abs, hip abductors, quadriceps, glutes, calves

Headings:

Practice this first in your front room or lawn until you are positive about your capacity. Standing up tall, step to the right with your right foot and carry your pass by walking to meet your right. Keep evading to the right multiple times.

Shift course and presently step to one side with your left foot. Carry your right foot to meet your left and keep avoiding the left multiple times.

Rehash multiple times.

To step up: Once you are confident in this move, you can rehearse this on your strolls outside. Turn sideways while strolling and avoid for 10 stages in a single course prior to changing to the opposite side. Make sure to constantly keep your head confronting the bearing you are moving.

Observe: Sidestepping is a regular ability that you use at home, in stores, and anyplace there are individuals around. Try not to peer down at your feet. Rather gaze directly ahead or toward the path you are moving.

Stroll on Heels and Toes

Length of activity: 30 seconds

All out time: brief 30 seconds

Regions dealt with: abs, hip flexors, calves

Headings:

Make certain to heat up your legs and feet by strolling regularly for five minutes prior to beginning this activity. You can clutch a ledge or enroll the assistance of a companion on the off chance that you want added help.

Walk gradually forward behind you with your toes taken off the ground. Stroll for 10 stages.

Stroll forward regularly for 10 stages.

Presently, gradually stroll on your toes with your heels taken off the ground. Stroll for 10 stages.

Rehash twice.

Observe: If your calves or feet are beginning to squeeze, enjoy some time off, and do just a large portion of the means. Increment how much advances just when you are agreeable.

Crisscross Walking

Length of activity: 1 moment

Absolute time: 5 minutes

Regions chipped away at: abs, hips, quadriceps, hamstrings, calves

Bearings:

This activity requires directional movements to expand your balance while strolling. You can set up two cones six feet separated and stroll in a figure eight example around the cones. Rehash multiple times.

Then again, you can stroll in a crisscross example on a way or walkway. Stroll forward at a point towards the right half of the way, then, at that point, stroll forward towards the left half of the way. Crisscross this way and that across the way a few times.

Observe: Because strolling in a serpentine example implies a shift in course, your balance will be tested. Keep your center muscles drawn in as you walk.

As referenced before, the top purposes behind getting into a strength-training program is to get more grounded and fabricate and keep up with bulk, the two of which can prompt other wellbeing and stylish advantages over the long haul. While there are numerous strength-training programs out there, there is one likeness they all share - basically the ones deserving at least moderate respect - are the center lifting exercises. These center exercises are a staple of the best strength-training projects of a considerable lot of the world's top jocks and power lifters essentially in light of the fact that they work best as far as making individuals more grounded and stronger. They consume the most calories which likewise makes them a staple of numerous wellness models' training programs!

The center lifting exercises any great strength-training project ought to incorporate are the squats, deadlifts, upward presses, and seat presses. Regardless of whether you have different exercises separated from these, you can develop huge fortitude and bulk on the grounds that these are what we call multi-joint or compound exercises. Recollect our conversation in the past part on what makes for a decent strength-training program? On the off chance that you do, you'd recall that these sorts of exercises are a fundamental piece of any strong strength-training program.

For what reason would they say they are so critical for any genuine strength-training program? This is on the grounds that these are exercises that utilize something other than one muscle bunch to lift as well as balance the loads. Dissimilar to a chest segregation work out, similar to hand weight flyes, which just work the chest, the seat press works the chest and different muscles, similar to the rear arm muscles, the center muscles, and somewhat, the shoulder muscles for soundness and balance. Additionally, dissimilar to a disconnection workout, for example, the leg press machine that mainly works the thighs, a hand weight squat works the thighs, the hamstrings, the calves, the lower back, and abs.

As an amateur, begin by performing 3 arrangements of 10 to 12 repetitions for each set per workout. Why 10 to 12 redundancies, and why just 3 sets? On the off chance that you're a novice and haven't had any weight-lifting experience, your muscles need to foster muscle memory, especially lifting utilizing appropriate structure. Assuming you focus on under 10 redundancies for each set, this implies you'll lift loads that might be excessively weighty for you as a still novice figuring out how to foster the propensity for legitimate structure. Why 3 sets as it were? This is on the grounds that your muscles are as yet not prepared to do extremely focused energy or responsibilities as a novice. Following 3 to a half year of working out with

3 arrangements of 10 to 12 reps for every set, you can begin going lower on the reiterations, higher on the weight, and higher in the quantity of sets up to 5 for each activity. You can likewise begin consolidating other weight-lifting exercises, including detachment exercises, to your program to enhance your center lifting exercises for significantly more noteworthy strength and mass increases.

CHAPTER 7

STRETCHING WORKOUT.

S omething we have dealt with in life is that not all things are advantageous. It could have taken us 60+ years to sort this one out, however essentially, we're onto something great.

As you arrive at 60 and head past its boundaries, you will be immersed with stunts, hacks, and procedures for expanding your childhood, deceiving the clock, and putting your best self forward. These current themselves via online media stages, through instant messages from companions who got them from companions (and their companions, etc) and even TV adverts. Something we were unable to help, however, notice was that such large numbers of the advertising ploys (and that is actually what they are, coincidentally) focused on us were/are centered around alternate routes and worth less methodologies. Hell, we even experienced a cream produced using snail sludge that professes to switch the indications of maturing in individuals 60 or more.

It's the ideal opportunity for one of those rude awakenings. Not all that you experience offering the mystery (or way) to everlasting youth and spryness is honest. Truth be told, large numbers of them need esteem. If somebody (or an advert) lets you know that it's the speediest and least demanding method for weighting misfortune, smooth, without wrinkle skin, an assuaged entrail (instead of a touchy one), and sparkling muscles protruding in regions they never swell before in your childhood, you're being deceived. You're only a cash hotspot for whoever is behind those vacant guarantees.

What works? Difficult work, work. Time and exertion work. Stretching works. Since it is valuable to you, it won't be a stroll in the park. It will require some work. So, move back from trend 60+ers diet plans, quit purchasing those gimmicky "do this for 5 minutes per day" body change contraptions, and spotlight on something truly useful to you. The best spot for anybody of our age to begin is with stretching. In section one, we previously covered the many advantages of stretching. Presently it is the ideal opportunity for us to talk about these advantages in a smidgen more detail.

One of the principal things we really want to specify is that it is fundamental to keep a scope of movement inside your joints. On the off chance that you don't, the muscles abbreviate and turn out to be tight - and trust us, that is awkward. Recall that companion of our own who hurt her shoulder while coming up from her seat on a flight? In the event that you're not ready to invest the energy now, that could be you. You could guiltlessly reach up to say change a light, and out of nowhere, the aggravation and strain flows through your body, prompting a very long time of restoring medicines that seldom accomplish the results you expect.

So, stretching keeps your muscles sound, solid, and adaptable. Very much stretched muscles are prepared when you want them, and even better, they're not inclined to injury when you truly do require them. Stretching is a simple venturing stone for greater development. Along these lines, assuming you want to turn out to be more dynamic once more, executing a customary stretching routine ought to be your initial step. However, obviously, assuming you have any previous circumstances that have made exercise and stretching inconceivable throughout the long term, it is ideal to talk with your doctor before you begin getting dynamic.

Who cares About Stretching Anyway?

With the present chatter about stretching, there will undoubtedly be a couple of cynics who have their questions. You could ask why stretching is significant for somebody north of 60 when you appear to have scraped by fine and dandy without it for such a long time. The thing is, you have recently squeezed by. You haven't flourished, and we need you to flourish. You without a doubt feel the niggling, throbbing painfulness that accompanies age, and fortunately they are reversible. All trust isn't lost! All There's justifications for why 60+ can be your greatest years yet. To give you something to go on, how about we see four designated ways stretching can uphold dynamic maturing, and keep troublesome muscle snugness and throbs under control.

Stretching soothes lower back torment and decreases

side effects of joint pain. Back torment has an approach to surprising us in our 60s. Lower back torment, specifically, is frequently the aftereffect of spinal stenosis, Osteoarthritis, or the one we as a whole prefer not to concede, conveying additional weight. On the off chance that your additional delicate to advanced age as certain individuals is, the ligament between the joints might decline and cause extra agony (this is really stenosis). Osteoarthritis is additionally nothing to laugh at. It's an agonizing infection that influences 33% of 60+ers. While stretching can't switch the circumstances influencing your lower back, it will go quite far to diminishing the torment, further developing adaptability, lightening joint firmness, and expanding your scope of movement. You could be saying your back aggravation and affectionate goodbye just by subscribing to normal stretching.

Stretching decreases the gamble of falling. Being 60+ can feel like fighting with the climate around you. Everything appears to need to push you over, trip you up, or see you rushing through the air. Actually, it's not actually advanced age to fault - it's your absence of balance and soundness. While general imbalance accompanies age, you can really chip away at being more adaptable, strong and balanced. Research shows that adaptability and scope of movement are basic to making the soundness important to decrease the gamble of falling. To be much less unstable on your feet, improving and holding adaptability in the hamstrings and quadriceps is fundamental. These muscles straightforwardly sway your static balance. One more region that you really want to keep versatile and solid are the hip joints since they likewise sway static balance. Before you ask, static balance is the point at which you are stopping. Then again, dynamic balance is having the option to keep up with balance and be tough on your feet while you're moving. Stretching strengthens the muscles, expands adaptability and further develops scope of movement - everything expected for better balance. So lengthy slip and fall occurrences! You're before long going to be solidly planted on your feet!

Stretching upholds a great stance. Presently that your 60+, you need to pay for the transgressions of your

114

childhood. Sit back and relax; we're not going to delve too profoundly into your past! Perhaps the greatest result is that 60+ers pay is an unfortunate stance because of a day-to-day existence spent slouched over a work area, or more regrettable yet, a cell phone. Presently, as a 60+er, out of nowhere you're donning a slouched back or can drop down in seats. What's the deal? The absolute first thing you totally need to know is that unfortunate stance packs the spine, which thus causes bothersome lower back torment. With every day stretching, stance can improve, and torment can (and will) decrease. With ordinary and committed stretching (that is doing the right stretches), you can altogether expand adaptability and slacken tight tendons, muscles, and ligaments.

Stretching further develops energy and blood flow. While doing our examination for this book, we ran over some really fascinating data on the job of blood stream (or course, as you could call it) on the body. For example, did you have any idea that having unfortunate flow can prompt laziness, joint agony, hemorrhoids, poor mental clarity and, surprisingly, more extreme circumstances, for example, phlebitis, cardiovascular

115

failures and strokes? Blood stream additionally conveys oxygen to all your crucial organs, so assuming your bloodstream is lazy, the odds are good that your organs aren't working at their maximum capacity.

Stretching is known to help blood stream and send solid oxygenated blood all through the body. This prompts more energy, advanced organs, and less possibility of succumbing to the circumstances referenced previously. Stretches that assist with supporting flow incorporate arm swings, shoulder circles, jumps, leg swings, and squats. While stretching gets your dissemination rolling, it likewise builds adaptability and expands scope of movement - it's an incredible all-rounder!

Stretching Tips and Advice

While we investigate explicit stretches you should zero in on when your 60+ in Chapter Six, we might want to share a couple of tips and guidance for safe stretching the correct way underneath. How about we stretch!

Zero in on significant muscle gatherings. You should focus on stretching significant muscle gatherings, for example, your calves, hips, lower back, thighs, neck, and shoulders. Guarantee that you stretch each side of your body, zeroing in on stretching muscles and joints that you regularly use.

Try not to bob. For reasons unknown, many individuals have an internal inclination to ricochet while stretching. You can definitely relax - we have all made it happen. All things being equal, stretch utilizing a smooth development, expanding your muscles outward without ricocheting. Bobbing may feel ideal to begin with, yet it's a dependable method for harming or straining your muscles. By abstaining from ricocheting, you guarantee a smooth and delicate development. Assuming you feel any sharp torments while stretching, stop right away.

Hold your stretch. In all honesty, stretching is a gradual cycle. There's no race included, so you're treating it terribly assuming you end up racing through them. All things considered, inhale regularly and hold each stretch for around 20 to 30 seconds prior to continuing on.

Try not to focus on torment. Hope to feel pressure while you're stretching, not torment. Stretching should feel great to your muscles, back, and joints. If stretching is difficult, dial down to where you don't feel any aggravation, then, at that point, hold the stretch. Now and again a full stretch is unimaginable, particularly in the event that you've been dormant for quite a while. Just stretch to the extent that you can without feeling torment until you have greater adaptability in the muscle. It creates over the long haul - simply show restraint toward yourself.

When you start a stretching schedule, make a big difference for it. Like most things you attempt to do throughout everyday life, you must be predictable with stretching to see long haul results. Stretching is something you need to do each and every day. The more you stretch, the more straightforward it will get. In any case, in the event that you stop half a month in, you will observe it trying to begin once more.

How Does Stretching Work?

How does stretching really function? We should

discuss the physiology of stretching. To lay it out plainly, stretching includes the muscles and joints cooperating. At this point, you are most likely mindful that ligaments connect muscles to the bones. Muscles can make the body move by connecting with the bones, ligaments and tendons. All things considered, the bones, ligaments, and tendons don't have similar capacity as the muscles. Compression and unwinding of the muscle change the strain on the joints, which prompts development of the body. Stretching is to ensure when the muscle, joints, ligaments, and so forth, are performing work and getting, the strain between them doesn't cause injury.

This extremely improved on clarification of how stretching functions lets us know that adaptability and scope of movement depend on your muscles, ligament and joints. At the point when these are cooperating, you will see a distinction in your knees, lower legs, and hips. They easily twist farther than previously, expand like never before, and be without torment at the same time. One motivation behind why it is significant to stretch similarly on the two sides is that drained muscles will make the restricting gatherings of muscles work more diligently. You will see muscle exhaustion on the opposite side of your body and the failure of the encompassing muscles to safeguard the joints from more extreme wounds in the event that your stretching isn't equivalent on the two sides.

Work on Your Quality of Life

We should discuss your personal satisfaction briefly. Most 60+ers would rather not become a weight to people around them. They likewise don't have any desire to spend each waking moment stuck to the couch since everything simply appears to be a mind-boggling physical exertion.

Tragically, you will be a weight or conceivably stable on the off chance that you don't invest energy staying in shape and dynamic. Your energy and wellness levels won't normally improve as you progress in years. They will absolutely deteriorate. Be that as it may, by stepping in with some solid stretching, you can intrude on the descending twisting of going downhill and fixed. Stretching is certifiably not a handy solution;

however, it is the key to an existence of 60+ where you can twist and stretch for things effectively, convey your own food, and bear less of a throbbing painfulness en route.

We talk from our very own experience when we let you know that stretching makes you more steady, more ready (to do as such numerous things!), and defter. Only a couple of years prior, we weren't playing the games we love or taking off for a Sunday morning run. Ordinary exercises accompanied the gamble of injury, and we feared the throbs, agonies and strains after a high-energy morning with the grandchildren. Everything that has changed for us, and to be very legitimate, everything began with a basic day by day stretching schedule.

We've as of now covered the advantages of beginning your day with a couple stretches, yet it's a subject definitely worth returning to. Before we move onto Chapter Three, we should recap every one of the manners by which you stand to profit from a standard stretching schedule.

The Benefits of Starting Your Day with Basic Stretches

1. Stretching launches blood dissemination, which initiates the body and psyche with a new surge of supplements and oxygen. Simultaneously, muscles that have been very still for a long time are gradually slipping into activity. The increase in oxygenated blood will likewise provide you with a nice explosion of energy for the afternoon.

2. Stretching strengthens muscles and further develops adaptability, which works on your stance, loosens up muscles, and warms them up.

3. Stretching offers back torment its walking orders! Stretching facilitates strain in the neck and back, assisting with lightning torment while strengthening the muscles simultaneously.

A couple of years back, we probably wouldn't have accepted that our 60+ lives could look so changed. Who realized that accomplishing something as basic as stretching could change all that we expected in advanced age. What's more, since we started acquainting ourselves with the idea of stretching with more 60+ers around us, we have seen critical upgrades in their lives as well. The test lies in getting everything rolling. You don't need to place in hours consistently. You can zero in on placing in only 20 minutes out of each day, four to five days per week. Keep this awake for 21 days, and afterward conclude what you think and feel. We're willing to wager you'll can't escape stretching and delighting in the physical advantages. Whenever we got everything rolling, we zeroed in exclusively on completing a couple stretches each day and afterward consistently before bed. Following half a month, we both began seeing our unquestionably expanded energy levels; thus, we chose to take it up a level (or three, in fact). We began slowly, however presently we play sports, go for runs, stay aware of the grandchildren and have a newly discovered pizzazz!

It's Time to Stretch!

We've spoken sufficiently with regards to how stretching functions, the advantages, and why you really want to begin today. Presently, it's an ideal opportunity to consider which stretches are best for you. Regardless, we have chosen seven of the stretching practices we completely appreciated when we initially began stretching. We call these our personal satisfaction stretches on the grounds that they truly worked effectively on our own! Assuming you at any point get to meet us (wouldn't so be extraordinary!), you will rapidly find that we're a couple that likes to try to do what we say others should do. Each activity included beneath is a standard that launched our direction back to wellbeing - yet used today.

CHAPTER 8
BASIC RULES FOR A HEALTHY DIET FOR PEOPLE OVER 60.

Whenever you have arrived at the expected degree of carbs and kept up with it for at least seven days, your body will consume its stores of glucose and begin initiating center ketogenic processes. The liver then, at that point, separates put away fat into a couple of particles, unsaturated fat, and glycerol. Unsaturated fats make it workable for the body to make ketones in any case, while the glycerol fills in for the glucose in explicit occurrences where the ketones can't give what the body needs. One such piece of the body is the cerebrum as it makes energy through what is known as gluconeogenesis.

While attempting to in a real sense dissolve the fat off your body is an extraordinary beginning, there are various extra advantages with regards to staying in the ketogenic state for a delayed timeframe. In addition, the more extended the state perseveres, the more articulated the beneficial outcomes become.

Works on a safe framework: beside how it is equipped for treating your general degree of appetite, the ketogenic state is known to drastically decrease the probability of various significant medical problems, beginning with every one of the kinds of disease that are known to benefit from glucose straightforwardly. While solid cells can undoubtedly change to consuming ketones for energy, disease cells are not that fortunate which implies they become altogether more leisurely than they in any case would when denied of their essential food source.

Changing to the keto diet is likewise ideal with regards to advancing cerebrum wellbeing for a very long time. The most significant of these is the way that after the keto diet is nearer to the manner in which early people probably ate which implies it is more in accordance with the sort of fuel that the mind is normally used to consuming. This, thus, makes it feasible for the cerebrum to keep working at its greatest limit with respect to longer than would somehow or another be the situation.

While it is actually the case that the cerebrum expects glucose to work appropriately, this is most certainly the situation of possibly having an overdose of something that is otherwise good. In the event that the mind gets a lot of glucose consistently, over the long haul it will foster a higher resilience which implies that it should work more enthusiastically to produce similar outcomes. Assuming that left untreated this can prompt a condition of glucose hardship which can ultimately prompt dementia. Using glycerol as a substitution for glucose can then make it more straightforward for the cerebrum to work in the long haul without stressing over these sorts of antagonistic impacts, implying that almost certainly, debasement will happen.

Diminishes hunger: past essentially assisting you with consuming fat all the more successfully, following a keto diet is additionally an incredible method for getting more fit for various different reasons, beginning with the way that leftover in ketosis is really demonstrated to assist you with residual inclination full after a dinner far longer than would somehow be the situation. This is basically because of the way that fat is more challenging to process than carbs which implies your body won't start to convey signals saying it is eager until all that has been totally handled.

Furthermore, while you can expect some carb desires during the early piece of ketosis, you will observe that after you make it past this obstacle you will actually want to eliminate food from your musings more effectively than previously. This is on account of a helpful chemical known as cholecystokinin which is the regular counter to ghrelin, the chemical answerable for letting you know when you are eager. Cholecystokinin is made by the body when food is traveling through the digestive organs, however on the off chance that you are in ketosis, it will be made consistently all things considered. The expanded cholecystokinin creation will go on for the full time your body stays in a ketogenic state, and in any event, for a couple of days after you have left it.

Additionally, other than helping you look and to have an improved outlook, the keto diet will likewise assist you with feeling fuller, longer and in the wake of eating a more modest serving of food. This is a characteristic result of a high fat and protein diet as both of these will stay with you significantly longer than sugars will. Likewise, after you have entered a ketogenic state then your body will normally begin by consuming instinctive fat which is basically fat that is put away in the midriff. All things considered; a ketogenic state makes a situation where your opportunity of coronary illness diminishes while your degree of positive cholesterol increases. It is additionally known to decrease your gamble of stroke and different other cardiovascular issues.

Choose the right keto plan
Low-carb, high-fat

Improved weight reduction - by forestalling the aggregation of sugars in the body, ketogenic consumes less calories and drives down insulin creation. This constrains our body to go through fat put away all over.

In any event, when you are dozing, the body will be consuming fat for its requirements! The fat that is being singed isn't simply the fat you ate yet in addition put away muscle versus fat. This will be a colossal assistance in decreasing weight.

It assists you with dealing with your yearning better - fat is an exceptionally fulfilling and filling supplement and ketone bodies decrease craving so you will feel undeniably less appetite than previously. Truth be told, there are times when you may very well neglect to eat! This is the most interesting piece of a ketogenic diet. You are roused to proceed with your endeavors as you are not battling with cravings for food.

It utilizes put away muscle versus fat as fuel - keto achieves a state where your body perceives your body fats as a practical wellspring of energy and continues to use it, in this manner creating the ketone bodies for fuel. In any case, other than focusing on the way that your body fats are being scorched while being in ketosis, getting your framework to perceive those equivalent fats as fuel additionally empowers you to go on discontinuous fasting a lot more straightforward and speedier.

It empowers quicker and better recuperation from work out - one of the vitally known foundations for those hurts and crudeness after an exercise is basically your body's fundamental irritation. That, thus, has been connected causally to the presence of free revolutionaries framed because of high measures of sugar admission. On a low carb high fat ketogenic diet, your body's fundamental irritation will go down because of lesser carbs and accordingly lower glucose levels

It diminishes and directs the degrees of insulin - on a higher carb diet, our body would basically be exposed to spikes of insulin each time our glucose levels spike because of the need to deal with it. That sugar must head off to some place!

Wholesome ketosis works with the decrease of insulin levels simply on the grounds that your body has brought down degrees of glucose through lesser utilization of carbs. The insulin spikes are likewise dealt with when your body switches over to ketones as the essential wellspring of fuel.

Anybody needing to lose and keep up with their body weight, anybody needing to turn out to be more vigorous and dynamic, any individual who needs to oversee troublesome ailments like diabetes and more can go ahead and get everything rolling on ketogenic eats less carbs.

Notwithstanding, there are a few distinct contraindications to keto counts calories. We are concerned essentially individuals who have a past filled with kidney, liver or gallbladder breakdown issues. The gallbladder is the store of stomach related catalysts fabricated from the liver used to separate fat. Subsequently these two organs can be supposed to be genuinely significant for somebody needing to get going on the high fat based ketogenic diet. Here are a few circumstances that appropriate a doctor's endorsement prior to getting going on a keto diet:

- impeded liver working

- gallbladder related issues

- pregnancy and lactation

- history of kidney disappointment

- disabled fat absorption

- history of pancreatitis

- gastric detour a medical procedure

While the recently referenced above are a couple of conditions recorded where it is empowered that you see your doctor prior to getting going on a keto diet, if it's not too much trouble, go ahead and converse with the person in question in any case prior to leaving on your keto venture assuming you feel awkward. Proficient exhortation is generally something to be thankful for.

Ketogenic slims down are not to be taken as simple weight control plans yet an implanted piece of your new way of life. The viability and accomplishment of ketogenic diets will be felt, experienced, and seen just when you track down the discipline and mental fortitude to venture out forward.

As may be obvious, ketogenic diets can assist you with getting a great deal of advantages, and it is those benefits which will move you along when you take up this adjustment of diet. Envision having the option to see the scales report back your deficiency of weight inside half a month of being in ketosis, and having the option to keep it there in the ideal reach unafraid of bounce back. What about visiting your cardiologist after a supported drive-in ketosis and having him take you off prescriptions for hypertension and other metabolic issues? These are not fantastical thoughts and can be accomplished with responsibility.

A decent ketogenic diet will assist you with getting your energy from fats, a more economical energy source than carbs.

Weight reduction and muscle gain are the most apparent advantages of fasting. In any case, there are various advantages connected with discontinuous fasting past fat copying and muscle gain. In the past, fasting periods were alluded to as detoxification, refinement and different equivalent words for purifying the body. The essential thought is to abstain from eating nourishment for an exact period. Likewise, discontinuous fasting is totally different from eating less junk food, which is troublesome and can be costly as well.

There are many advantages of irregular fasting, the most significant of which are the accompanying:

• irregular fasting, when matched with spotless, natural, nutritious food eaten with some restraint and the reward of actual work, can bring about consistent, steady weight reduction that stays off!

• support and expected increase of fit bulk

• further developed digestion, which is helpful to mind wellbeing, digestion is the name for the vital synthetic responses that occur in your cells.

• further developed ketone creation. Ketone is a compound that safeguards the mind when there is a decline of free glucose.

• further develops craving control - irregular fasting permits you to perceive among mental and actual yearning

• may lessen manifestations of melancholy by

managing insulin and glucose levels.

- upgrades execution on memory tests in the old

- decreases oxidative pressure, harm, and aggravation in the body

- hormonal rebalancing - insulin levels and insulin obstruction; leptin; ghrelin additionally, human development chemical increments and works with fat consuming and muscle gain

- expanded endurance - competitors who practice on an unfilled stomach have encountered more energy and endurance. It is trusted that the mix of fasting and practicing triggers inner impetuses that power the breakdown of sugars and fat into energy, without forfeiting bulk.

- assists with food desires - as your leptin and ghrelin levels reset to your discontinuous fasting plan, old triggers to eat specific food sources at specific times will be eradicated.

- quality security - connected with life span and insurance against illnesses, remembering promising examination for malignant growth

Indeed, Keto is valuable and indeed, it has a great deal of advantages, however it is no small thing, thus, it should be drawn nearer with alertness. Here are a few hints you should remember prior to leaving on Keto.

Utilize plans you can trust

Keto includes a ton of supper arranging and this single stage is the place where many individuals fail to understand the situation. Your dinners are not generally permitted to be indiscreet and you should note all that goes into your mouth. Assuming you are setting out on a Keto diet, you should utilize plans you can trust. The plans should be advantageous, safe, and flavorful. Keto ought not take out the satisfaction in your dinners.

You might require a specialist

Assuming that you have disapproved of glucose, insulin levels or diabetes, counsel your primary care physician prior to leaving on Keto. Try not to roll out any dietary improvements as extensive as Keto to your eating regimen without first illuminating your primary care physician. The individual in question is in the best situation to direct you appropriately. See your PCP.

It will be hard right away

Keto is no stroll in the park. Be that as it may, individuals progress forward with the way of Keto notwithstanding the underlying trouble in light of the fact that the outcomes are obvious after a brief time. Whenever you launch Keto, you might experience the ill effects of low glucose, laziness, and obstruction, However, they will all wear off in a couple of days assuming you are strict with regards to it.

Would Keto be able to have incidental effects?

Indeed. Keto can have aftereffects. Keto can have negative aftereffects in the event that it is wrongly finished. Keto eliminates carbs and replaces them with fat. Notwithstanding, in the event that the substitution isn't enough completed, a great deal of negative secondary effects might happen. Therefore, it is critical to start the Keto diet outfitted with the right data and plans which are totally remembered for this book.

In the event that you don't utilize quality feast plans and plans, you'll need supplements that your body needs. With Keto, you should not need proteins thus, your suppers should be arranged.

Step by step instructions to arrive at ketosis

Arriving at the condition of ketosis isn't so clear for some individuals. To successfully arrive at ketosis, there are a few stages you should take.

Eat the right food-Ketosis depends a ton on what you eat. To arrive at ketosis, you really want to initially eliminate the carbs you take in. Furthermore, you really want to take in significantly more fats in your weight control plans. Notwithstanding, you should simply take in any fat, you should try to take in sound fat. Taking in unfortunate fats can hurt more than great.

Work out to productively arrive at ketosis, you should try to work out. It doesn't need to be serious, in any case, long strolls, containers, trekking, and different activities can assist your body with arriving at ketosis.

Attempt irregular fasting-Some individuals join

discontinuous fasting with ketosis. The explanation is that, as you progress, your cravings for food are diminished extraordinarily and you will find irregular fasting simple. Indeed, in any event, when you don't plan to, you'll wind up making it happen. It is certainly not obligatory yet on the off chance that you are utilizing ketosis to shed pounds, irregular fasting is an extraordinary reward.

Taking bunches of leafy foods Fruits and vegetables for bites will keep your body solid and assist with renewing your skin.

Incorporate coconut oil in your eating routine Coconut is obligatory to arrive at ketosis. Coconut oil contains sound fat. It assists the body with arriving at ketosis and contains four kinds of MCTs. It is perhaps the best apparatus for inciting ketosis.

Keto Compared to Other Diets

Once more, the keto diet isn't the main eating regimen that exists in the realm of wellness and wellbeing. You are managing the cost of a wide scope of choices and systems that you can decide to embrace for yourself. This sort of assortment and variety inside the business of counting calories is continuously going to be great. Thus, individuals will be ready to track down the eating routine that best suits their very own necessities and their own ways of life. What's more, assuming you are one who is considering embracing the keto diet for your own life, then, at that point, you will need to know exactly the way in which it looks at different other options.

What's more, that will fill in as the point for this part. You will be given a brief look into what the keto diet truly is and the way that it piles up comparative with the other well-known weight control plans out there available. This sort of relative examination would have the option to complete two things. One, it will permit you to accumulate points of view on the eating regimen industry and the assortment of choices that are accessible for you to attempt. Also, two, it will offer you a more educated assessment and a more grounded resolve for anything diet plan you truly do ultimately decide to take on for yourself later on.

A Case for Keto Being the Best Diet Plan Out There

It is actually the case that there are for sure endless eating routine plans out there available, and it would be too self-important to even consider saying that the keto diet is awesome among them all. Notwithstanding, it would be reasonable to say that the keto diet is the best one for you by and by assuming it ends up serving your requirements and your objectives all the more actually.

The keto diet is a low-carb diet that is intended to place the human body into an uplifted ketogenic state, which would definitely prompt more articulated fat consumption and weight reduction. It is a genuinely open eating routine with a great deal of keto-accommodating food sources being promptly accessible in commercial centers at somewhat reasonable costs. It isn't actually an eating routine that is held uniquely for the well-off and world class.

Taking everything into account, there is only no denying how effective a keto diet can be for an individual who needs to lose an extraordinary measure of weight in a solid and controlled way. The keto diet additionally authorizes discipline and accuracy for the specialist by consolidating large scale counting and food journaling to guarantee precision and responsibility in the eating routine. There are no outside factors that can affect how successful this diet can be for you. Everything is all inside your control.

Furthermore finally, it's a genuinely supportable eating regimen plan, considering that it doesn't actually think twice about flavor or assortment. Certainly, there are a lot of limitations. In any case, there are a ton of choices and workarounds that can help fight off desires. Assuming this multitude of standards and reasons concern you and your own life, then, at that point, it would be safe to say that the keto diet is the best one for you.

What Sets Keto Apart from Others?

In any case, how precisely does keto stack facing other eating routine plans out there? Indeed, in the event that your motivation for counting calories is weight reduction, it would be judicious to investigate different eating regimens that are like the keto diet's objectives of promoting weight reduction and fat consumption. You should acquire a superior comprehension of these weight control plans and why the keto diet would most likely still be the better one for you. The three weight control plans that are generally normally contrasted with the keto diet as far as food creation and actual impacts are Atkins, paleo, and Whole30.

Atkins

The Atkins and keto counts calories are so comparable as in the two of them advance intense usage of fats, moderate utilization of protein, and insignificant utilization of carbs. Regularly, while on Atkins, an individual's common eating regimen would be made out of 60% fat, 30% protein, and 10% starches. This is as yet a moderately negligible carb structure in any event, when you think about the keto breakdown of 75% fat, 20% protein, and 5% carbs.

The issue with Atkins isn't actually found in the higher sugar utilization. It's generally found in the raised utilization of protein. Any abundance of protein that the body doesn't go through for muscle building or fix is changed over into glucose. Furthermore, that glucose will be utilized for energy rather than the put away fats that you can have, therefore making the metabolic pace of your body slower. The keto diet actually offers you the protein advantages of building and fixing muscles without compromising the advantages of ketosis simultaneously.

Paleo

The paleo diet is one that is acquiring immense prevalence in the contemporary wellness industry. It comes from the concentrated dietary acts of the Paleolithic period, which was reliant upon the agrarian arrangement of food apportioning and creation. It is an eating regimen that centers entirely around entire food sources that are liberated from any handling. Food things like wheat, grains, dairy, vegetables, handled sugars, handled oils, corn, handled fat, and so forth are restricted. It centers around the maximum usage of meats and non-bland vegetables.

Like the keto diet, the paleo diet likewise turns out to be a low-carb diet that underlines a higher utilization of fats and proteins. Notwithstanding, it doesn't actually restrict the quantity of starches or calories that an individual could take consistently. It's an eating routine arrangement that centers completely around the piece of food without its amount, and that can be dangerous for many individuals who have unmistakable actual organization objectives.

Whole30

Whole30 is basically a stricter rendition of the paleo diet. It is an eating routine arrangement that is basically organized as a thirty-day program of severe eating under paleo standards. It totally dispenses with the utilization of handled food sources, boring vegetables and sugars, sugars, dairy items, vegetables, and that's only the tip of the iceberg. When the thirty-day time frame is finished, you are then encouraged to once again introduce specific nutrition types continuously in your eating regimen and see what sort of impact or effect these can have on you. This is the manner by which you will actually want to discover what sort of food you have an overall prejudice to.

Nonetheless, the Whole30 diet doesn't actually factor in large scale counting and calorie counting all things considered. That implies that individuals on the Whole30 diet are as yet powerless to putting on weight and getting fat regardless of the prohibitive idea of the eating routine.

These could be three instances of comparative dietary projects and approaches, and there are such countless different eating regimens out there that the keto diet can really measure up to. In any case, that would likely make for another book altogether. The point that this section is simply attempting to make and stress is that there are continuously going to be sure admonitions in any sort of dietary way of thinking. There will be advantages, and there will be cons also. The most ideal sort of diet isn't the one that everyone on the planet will track down achievement in. Rather, it's the one that will empower you to arrive at all your very own wellness objectives and dreams. Also, it would be exceptionally difficult to deny the way that the keto diet figures out how to do exactly that for such countless various types of individuals on the planet.

CONCLUSION

The ways that you take care of your body and the ways you stay active will dictate your quality of life and how good you will look. If you do not take care of your body, you might be 60 years old and look like you are sixty-five years old. But if you do good things for your body, you might be sixty-five years old and look like you are 60 years old. Age really is just a number. And even if you haven't been active in a long time, or ever, it is never too late to start on some sort of activity plan to increase the quality of your life.

I call it an activity plan because no one really wants to exercise, right? So, let's think of this as an activity plan or a workout routine, both of those are positive statements that say you care about your body and you want to fight the effects of growing older with everything you've got.

Once a woman crosses that 60-year mark, she begins losing one percent of her muscle each year. But muscle tone and fiber do not need to be lost with aging. With a proper workout, you can continue to build new muscle and maintain what you already have until you are in your nineties. And some of the exercises that you do for your muscles will help you build strong bones. This is especially important for women because losing the estrogen supplies in our bodies will cause us to lose bone mass faster than men do. This is when we are really at risk for developing osteoporosis.

And regular physical activity will help you to avoid developing that middle-age spread around the abdomen or to lose it if you already have it. Activity will help you to maintain a proper weight for your height and build which in turn will help you to avoid many, if not all, of the age-related, obesity-related diseases such as cardiovascular diseases and diabetes.

Physical activity comes in four main types. Each one should be done at least once or twice a week to ensure your body is getting the right mix of activity. The four main types of activity are:

- **Balance** – Older people lose their sense of balance. It is easy for an older person to fall and break something, like a hip. When you engage in activities that help you to maintain your sense of balance will help reduce the risk that you might fall and suffer a permanent injury.

- **Stretching** – As we age our muscles begin to lose their elasticity. This is part of why rolling out of bed in the morning gets more difficult as we get older. Stretching activities will help you to improve and maintain your level of flexibility which will help you to avoid injuries to your joints and muscles.

- **Cardiovascular/Aerobic** – These are also called endurance activities because you should be able to maintain them for at least ten minutes at a time. This key here is to get your heart working faster and you're breathing to be deeper. You should be working hard but still able to carry on a conversation. These activities will strengthen your heart and lungs which are, after all, very important muscles in your body.

- **Strength training** – We are not talking about

bodybuilding, but if you want to go for it. This will include working out with resistance bands or lifting weights. Either activity will help to build muscle.

While there are four separate categories of exercise that does not mean that you need to keep them strictly separated because many activities will encompass work in more than one area. You can lift light weights while doing balanced activities. Walking and swimming will build muscle strength and cardiovascular health. Yoga will improve balance and assist with building muscle strength and stretching. The key is to engage in seventy-five minutes of vigorous activity each week, or fifteen minutes five days each week; or you can get one hundred 60 minutes of moderate activity in five thirty-minute sessions each week.

And make sure that you design a plan that fits you. Remember that it is perfectly fine to change your routine as your needs change. Maybe, in the beginning, you will work on balance three days each week because you really need help with that. But after a few weeks, your balance has improved enough so that you can devote one of those days to strength training. This is your routine made just for you so make it work for you. And don't forget to get your doctor's okay before beginning any type of activity routine. He will most likely give you his blessings but it is always good to ask. He can also provide you with information on activities that are good for you personally.

One thing to note here, especially if you have not been active in a while, is not to begin a vigorous level of activity the same day you begin the keto diet. During the time your body is getting used to the diet and going through ketosis, you will not feel like indulging in a lot of extra activity and your workout routine will be doomed to failure. This journey is all about making you the best you possibly can so don't sabotage yourself in the first few weeks. If you really want to start your activities on day one of your diet then I recommend walking or bicycling. Either of these activities can be started slowly, so a gentle walk or bike around the neighborhood after dinner is a perfect activity.

If you can get out and join a class at a local senior center, YMCA, community college, or church then do that. You will meet new people, some in your age group, and you can all work together to create your new bodies. But taking a class will not be the best choice for everyone. So, we have included some basic exercises that can be done in the privacy of your home to get you started on the new lean you.

STRETCHING – Stretching activities are so important for older adults. These activities will also help you to improve your balance because you might find yourself standing or reaching in new and different ways.

Quad stretch – This is a simple exercise that can be done at home. Hold onto a chair or your partner for balance assistance if you need it. Then with the opposite hand lift the foot on that side behind you. Pull upward gently you can feel the beginning of a stretch in the front of your leg. As people get older, they may lean forward for balance and this muscle, the quad, can become shorter and less efficient over time. Hold this position steady for at least thirty seconds and repeat on the other side.

Hamstring stretch – This activity can be done on the sofa, the bed, or on the floor. Lay one leg in front of you and point your toes to the ceiling. Slowly fold your body over until you feel a stretching in the back of your leg and hold it for thirty seconds. NOTE: if you have recently had a hip replacement check with your doctor before doing this one.

Calf stretch – Place your hands on the wall and step back with one foot. The back foot should be flat on the floor and the front knee should be slightly bent. Then lean forward toward the wall until you feel a stretch in your calf muscle. Hold it for thirty seconds and repeat on the other leg.

BALANCING – Balancing activities are so important for older adults to reduce the risk of falls. Tai Chi and Yoga are both excellent activities for assisting with better balance. You can find DVDs, routines online, or classes taught by certified instructors. Just remember to work with your body and your current level of ability and don't try to do an advanced routine if you have never mastered a beginner routine. You will just be setting yourself up for failure and we are here to succeed. And keep in mind that flexibility activities also help with the effects of arthritis. While you will want to explore the different types of yoga before making a decision on the one that is best for you, here is a yoga pose that anyone can do at home and helps to wake the whole body in the morning.

Mountain Pose – Stand straight with your feet together. Pull in your stomach muscles as tight as you can and let your shoulders relax. Keep your legs strong but do not lock your knees. Breathe deeply and regularly in and out for ten breaths.

Strength Training – This activity is especially important for you to ensure you keep your muscles strong and healthy for the next phase of your life. You can do many strength training activities without weights, or for an extra challenge add some light hand weights.

Punching – This will strengthen your arms and shoulders and get your blood moving at the same time.

Stand straight with your feet apart slightly wider than your shoulders. Keep your stomach firm. Punch straight out with one fist and then the other for at least twenty repetitions.

Squat – This activity is great for strengthening the bottom and the thighs. This will help you to sit down – not fall down – and be able to rise from a seated position with ease and grace. Stand with your feet as far apart as your hips are wide to provide a stable stance. Push your bottom backward as you bend your knees. Your knees should never go out front further than your toes, and try to keep your weight over your heels. If you feel more secure this activity can be done in front of a chair in case you lose your balance and inadvertently sit down.

Cardiovascular/Aerobic – The purpose here is to engage in some activity that gets your heart pumping faster and your lungs expanding further. Swimming, walking, running, cycling, aerobics classes, dancing – all of these are great activities for getting the circulation going again. Just remember to begin slowly and pay attention to your body. In other words, if something hurts, stop. But make sure it really hurts. There is a difference between 'Wow I'm really out of shape because I haven't walked anywhere in a while' and 'My knee really hurts when I do that'. And any time you are ever in doubt seek medical attention.

Seated Activities – The body will deteriorate if it is not used. Maybe you really want to engage in physical activities but you really can't stand up for long enough to do anything meaningful. You can sit down and do many activities that are designed to get you back into the routine of regular movement. Here are a few options for you:

Marching – sit tall in your chair with your feet flat on the floor and your legs bent at a ninety-degree angle. Lift one foot and then the other, as though you are marching in the chair. Raise the knee up in the air and keep the knee bent.

Shoulder Press – Sit tall in your chair. You can hold a set of light weights or simply make your hands into fists. If you do not own weights and do not want to buy any you can also use canned items or full water bottles.

Raise your hands up into the air until your arms are straight and then lower them. Do these slowly so that your muscles will actually be doing the work.

Leg lifts – This activity will strengthen your quads, which is the muscle on the front of your leg. Strong quads are needed for walking upright. Sit tall in your chair with your knees bent at ninety degrees and your feet flat on the floor. Lift a foot up into the air and away from the chair slowly; let the muscle do the work. Hold the pose for five seconds and lower it. Repeat five times on each leg.

These are just a few of the activities that you can do to get yourself moving and help you in your weight loss and health goals. You are not too old to begin. You can find many routines on the internet so that you can use them alone in the privacy of your home. Remember to preview a routine before you pay for anything in case you do not like it. And many routines are offered free of charge. So do a bit of research and don't stop with one activity. Try to make your routine as varied as possible so that you will not get bored and soon you will have that body you want along with a healthier you.

Printed in Great Britain
by Amazon

81879880R00099